DANTE'S EIGHTH CIRCLE

Why Scientology's Narconon Must Be Stopped

DAVID E. LOVE

Dedicated to all who suffered injustice, to the many that have lost loved ones, and to those who had the courage to speak out and tell the truth. And to my father who passed away at age 39 when I was only nine — telling me: "Never start something if you're not going to finish it well, and never give up if it's for what's good and what's right." — Thanks Dad

Contents

	Contents	i
1	**The Road to Healing: Post-Traumatic Stress Disorder**	1
	A Cry for Help	6
	My Guardian Angel Arrives	13
2	**Vancouver to Scientology's Narconon in Quebec**	17
	Indoctrinated into Scientology	24
3	**Painful Beginnings in the Cult Compound**	27
	The Interrogations Begin	28
	A Quack Doctor and the Narconon Charlatans	32
4	**A Peek into Hell: the Stairway to Nightmares**	35
	Tarnishing Narconon's Reputation	38
	Messages to Me from a Young Mom	40
5	**A Cult of Paranoia**	43
6	**First Day in the Devil's Den of Hell**	47
7	**A Military Compound of Surveillance and Suffering**	51
	Punishment and Slavery	55
8	**Get Back in the Box**	59
9	**Held Against My Will**	65

	Accused of Cheating	66
10	Down the Rabbit Hole of Chaos	71
11	Hacking into Souls	77
12	Free Time Watching the Sickness	87
13	Roller-Coastering: Ups and Downs in Life Disaster	93
14	Confessions used to Attack their Enemy	99
	Another Battle Begins	101
15	A Cult of Quackery and Confusion	103
16	All Was Well in Hell: Slave Labour and Drama	109
17	Working for an Alien Cult: False Success Rate	119
18	My Dark Escape from a Cult of Paranoia	127
19	Help from Anonymous	139
20	Legal Battles and Educating the Community	143
	Ban the Doctor — a Milestone	147
	Narconon Trois-Rivières Shut Down by Health Agency	152
21	Pressing on into the United States and Ireland	155
22	Insane Fair Game: Dead Agent Attacks	165
	Online Attacks Continue	168
23	Spin-Doctoring Defamation Attacks	181
24	Roller Coaster 'Journey of Life' — What a Ride!	185
	An Event that Would Change My Life	186
	Time To Be My Own Boss	191
	The Death of a Baby	192
	Directing a Drug Rehab Center	193

Contents

    The Helicopter Ride 194

25 Man on Mission Possible   199

26 Human Rights Commission Verdict   205

27 Say No to Narconon at Trout Run   221
    The Decision 227
    Narconon in Canada Rejected 228

28 Full Circle: Love versus Goliath   231

Acknowledgements   243

References   245

Scientology Glossary   247

Introduction

This book is a memoir of specific life events, reliving emotions from being deceived that are difficult to admit or even to feel. It is an account of the altered states that trauma induces, which make it possible to survive a life-threatening event but impair the capacity to feel fear, and worse still, impair the ability to trust and love.

In the early 1990s I desperately wanted to attend law school at the University of British Columbia, Canada. I bought dozens of second hand law books — each being a page-turner of: "I want more!" Law school tuition was too costly for the years it would take while still having to support my family. So, I decided to take the Real Estate course through the University instead — it was only one year, and the study of contract law was intriguing. In my six year career as a Realtor and Sub-Mortgage Broker, drafting firm and binding contacts for clients was my specialty. Other Realtors approached me asking: "How did you put that deal together, David — can you show me how?" I loved my career. However, when I saw Realtors misrepresenting their property listings and/or walking a fine line towards fraud, I spoke up, reported it, and attended meetings with the Real Estate Board to have it stopped and discipline the offender.

Now, I'm here after witnessing fraud, misrepresentation, coercion, and human rights abuses by Scientology's Narconon drug rehab centers. I witnessed it, lived it every day, and knew I had to do something about it. For more than five years, I have been writing this book from memory, diarized notes, and victim accounts of their misery and the horrific trauma they suffered.

The book's title: DANTE'S EIGHTH CIRCLE is from a poem — "Dante's Inferno" about the nine circles of Hell — the 'Eighth' being FRAUD. That's

Dante's Eighth Circle

really what much of this book is about, all nine circles, but mostly the conscious fraud in the eighth circle.

    In my opinion, Scientology and their Narconon rehab centers are the image of fraud. The malicious damage caused to innocent victims is insidious. The fraud and those guilty of evil are surrounded by fraudulent advisers or evil counsellors. Of course, this book will touch on the "Fourth Circle — Greed" and the "Ninth Circle Treachery" — the latter being betrayal of special relationships and disconnection/shunning.

Foreward

To this very day I still wonder, "How could I have been so stupid?"

Stupid enough to fall for a cult of perpetual lies, fraud, and insidious practices of evil indoctrination.

I'm an intelligent, self-aware, educated, skilled person.

So how did I fall — hook, line and sinker — for the "drug treatment" scam known as Narconon, operated by the Church of Scientology to bilk its "students" of tens of thousands of dollars and to indoctrinate new members into "The Church"?

As I unravel the answer to this question for myself, I will explain my personal nightmare to you in vivid detail ... The hellish incidents of brainwashing and mind control, the lost sense of personal identity and a haunting period of post-traumatic stress. I hope that you might comprehend the pain, the nightmares, and sleepless nights, so you emerge armed with knowledge that can help you resist the pull of Narconon/Scientology, should it enter your life or the lives of anyone dear to you.

Chapter 1

The Road to Healing: Post-Traumatic Stress Disorder

The soul always knows what to do to heal itself. The challenge is to silence the mind. This is one of my finer quotations. —Caroline Myss

Many people think Post Traumatic Stress Disorder (PTSD) is reserved for our military heroes after returning home from wartime horrors. The truth is, all kinds of traumatic events can cause PTSD, and in some cases, CPTSD (Complex Post-Traumatic Stress Disorder), which is often endured by people who survive an experience with an abusive, mind-manipulating cult or group.

My involvement with the cult known as Scientology's Narconon changed something inside me to a degree that sometimes I doubt my mind will ever be the same. My negative experiences continued on for more than five years after my escape. I was informed by a therapist that the trauma I experienced can disrupt brain chemistry permanently. And I was one of the lucky ones who had the presence of mind to escape. I had only been in for eleven months. Countless others have been abused for years or decades and, if they come out alive, face years of recovery in far worse condition.

Please understand one overriding fact that I learned the hard way. Scientology's Narconon is a *Thriving Cult of Greed and Power*,[3] dictated by its current leader David Miscavige, who many allege is a narcissistic, psychotic, sociopath. I was battered around psychologically while in the cult and dealing with the resulting PTSD. When I began to speak out against Sci-

Dante's Eighth Circle

entology's Narconon, the attacks that followed, orchestrated by Scientology, were far worse.

As you travel with me on these pages, try to imagine what it would be like if your freedom of speech was taken away ... Think about not being allowed to show your emotions or pain. I was forced to abandon my freedom, hide the real me and convert to their cult belief system ... Scientology. Rooms were searched, books were taken away, and I dared not reveal my painful memories. Narconon executives scorned me and commanded I stay in present time.

We were very ill patients in a land of a new language to most of us. Narconon called us "students." Most, including myself, could not speak or understand the French language in Quebec. All the executives and many other staff were bilingual in French and English. They also spoke another language very foreign to me. They would use expressions such as "being at cause over life" and a raft of other meaningless jargon. And when the executives were talking among themselves in ears reach of students, they spoke in French.

I now have a much deeper respect for war veterans and prisoners of war, and I would never compare my experience to theirs. My experience inside this cult was tiny compared to what I imagine many soldiers had to endure. I can't even imagine some of the horror they went through and suffered from after returning home. But I can now understand how past traumatic events can carry forward and how they sculpt our minds and lead to severe anxiety and/or depression ... even suicide.

Being inside the Narconon compound was like living in a bubble void of information. We were cut off from the outside. For students, the internet was blocked to some websites (including Facebook) and newspapers were not allowed. We were all monitored day and night. I felt like a mouse in some weird experiment where, if the wrong door was pushed open, I would face brutal consequences.

I often flashback to a young lady being pulled out of a car, kicking and screaming: "No, no, no ... I don't want to go" as she was pulled by her arms with legs dragging on the ground on her way to the Withdrawal Detox Unit. She was in her mid-twenties or so. She was an adult who was being forced against her will. But, just like me, once there with no means to leave, she was stuck there for the duration. This young lady would suffer through

The Road to Healing: Post-Traumatic Stress Disorder

extreme emotions and physical pain.

It seemed like so many students who graduated the program, were then recruited to work as staff. I wondered if it would be the same for me. I was in a foreign land where they spoke a foreign language, and I shuddered at the thought of remaining on after the program to work as a staff member.

I remember, as if it was yesterday, two events at Narconon that convinced me to escape as soon as possible. The first event was when I discovered Narconon was a money-grabbing fraud, and the second was when I became aware of and believed it was an Alien worshipping Cult. Narconon was promoting a 76% success rate to desperate addicts and their family and promising their program was the best. In fact, 76% was closer to their program relapse rate and my eyes opened wider when I learned the truth about *Xenu*[1] and the Aliens in Scientology's doctrines.

Xenu is part of Scientology's secret "Advanced Technology" doctrines. He was the ruler of a Galactic Confederacy 75 million years ago, where the planets were overpopulated, containing an average population of 178 billion. Xenu was about to be deposed from power, so he paralyzed the aliens and loaded them into spacecraft and delivered them to earth.

My jaw dropped as I was reading this, but there was more ... much more.

It claimed that when they had reached planet earth, the paralyzed aliens were unloaded around the bases of volcanoes across the planet. Hydrogen bombs were then lowered into the volcanoes, blowing up the victims.

The now-disembodied alien souls, which Hubbard called "thetans," were blown into the air by the blast, killing all but a few. These became what are known as body thetans, which are said to be still clinging to and adversely affecting everyone. Only Scientologists who have performed the necessary steps to remove them through auditing sessions to the state of being 'CLEAR' experience total freedom.

This is when I realized why Narconon students, were called "Pre-Clears" (PCs) and subject to Scientology Training Routines and auditing sessions. It was the cult's indoctrination process to 'Clear' us of these little buggers clinging to us. In fact, the staff called our files "PC Folders." We were on our way to being 'Clear.'

---

[1] https://en.wikipedia.org/wiki/Xenu

And if that wasn't enough to twist someone's mind, there was the next step up to having 'Super Powers' ... being a Super Human Being. I could be an 'Operating Thetan' if I forked over huge sums and delivered my soul into the hands of an alien cult. It sent shivers down my spine and I could feel the hair itching on the back of my neck. It was time to leave.

Escaping Narconon would not be easy. I was being watched and suspected my internal emails were being monitored. On October 9, 2009, at 9:37 am, I received the following email from the 'head honcho' at Narconon:

> A bit of advice here ... for these kinds of personal communications, what I suggest is that you use your own personal email address (so nobody can hack in). My main concern is that in the past there has been staff that were able to "hack" in our data base somehow and check other staff emails (RJ and myself for sure). You were "a bit" nattery about Scott and you have to be careful around here because even the "walls have ears" ...

I contacted a person in Montreal who worked for the Canada Federal government who was willing to help. Whatever I needed to escape, they would provide. Over the next several days, I got all my ducks in a row. One hour and day at a time, I pretended to do something for Narconon, when in reality, I was in escape mode.

It was a dark winter evening in Quebec when the call came in. "David, I'm across from where you are in the mall parking lot. Where are you?" they asked. I replied, "Just give me six minutes and pick me up at the café across the road on the corner of the highway and 6th street." A few minutes later I was sitting in a car with someone I had never met, and we headed off down the highway to Montreal.

After I escaped, most days I felt on edge, sudden noises made me jump, and the nightmares kept coming back. They were more than real, and for good reason I suppose. One dream kept flashing back like the one I had so many times in my room at Narconon. I saw shades of darkness blending into cold black with distorted faces covered in blood ... some with wings hovering over me hissing. These nightmares were in the demonic realm. I had visions in my sleep like I had never seen before. This cult had invaded my mind. Other times, I would wake up soaking wet from dreaming of being chased ... the devil close behind.

The Road to Healing: Post-Traumatic Stress Disorder

At times, I felt like my life or the lives of others and my family were in danger, and that I had no control over what was happening to me. Only hours after I was escorted by police to pick up my belongings from Scientology's drug rehab, Narconon, I received a message on my Facebook wall from one of the executive directors who declared me an "Enemy." Being declared an "Enemy" was a "Suppressive Person (SP) Order." I was now subject to Scientology's "Fair Game." Stay with me here — Scientology has an arcane lexicon of terms fabricated by them. If you feel like you need a dictionary to keep up, there is a glossary at the end of this book. Bottom line, I had escaped the cult and now the cult was after me in a big way.

About six days after escaping Narconon Trois-Rivières, I showed up at the facility with a police escort and a CBC Radio Canada TV reporter and cameraman. This act drew the line in the sand — a 'them against me' battle against Scientology's Narconon that raged for six years and still does to this day.

This resulted in me being declared "Fair Game" by Scientology leadership. This meant (and still means), in Scientology's hierarchy, I "may be deprived of property or injured by any means by any Scientologist without any discipline of the Scientologist. May be tricked, sued or lied to or destroyed." In L. Ron Hubbard's confidential Manual of Justice he wrote:

> People attack Scientology. I never forget it, always even the score.
> — L. Ron Hubbard, MANUAL OF JUSTICE, 1959

He advocated using private investigators to investigate critics like me. "Hire them and damn the cost when you need to," he said. Hubbard instructed that when dealing with opponents, his followers should "always find or manufacture enough threat against them to cause them to sue for peace. Don't ever defend. Always attack and use 'black propaganda' to 'destroy the reputation or public belief in persons, companies or nations.' " — L. Ron Hubbard Policy Letter, 15 August 1960.

In 1965 Hubbard formulated the "Fair Game Law", which states how to deal with people who interfere with Scientology's activities, and in December of that year, Hubbard reissued the policy with additional clarifications to define the scope of Fair Game. He made it clear that the policy applied to non-Scientologists as well, declaring:

Dante's Eighth Circle

> The homes, property, places and abodes of persons who have been active in attempting to: suppress Scientology or Scientologists are all beyond any protection of Scientology Ethics, unless absolved by later Ethics or an amnesty … this Policy Letter extends to suppressive non-Scientology wives and husbands and parents, or other family members or hostile groups or even close friends.

Over the past few years, I have been threatened, physically pushed, followed, had emails hacked, and had "Dead Agent" letters sent out. The media, my employer, my friends, and even my young daughter received disgusting letters and links to websites that attacked my credibility. Scientology had declared war against me, and I would hit back ten-fold each time they attacked. I would use my laptop to fight back, exposing this insidious, dirty tricks cult for what it really was … unclean evil.

Many know me as a steadfast person who doesn't give up. I will press on no matter what, if driven by a just cause. But psychologically I was being worn down. I just couldn't grasp or understand what had happened and what was still happening to me. I began to have what I call "melt-downs" while writing and working on the computer — tears rolling down my face until I couldn't see the keyboard anymore. I was an emotional mess!

Some of the flash-backs to events at Narconon were reeling around in my mind, forcing me to experience the incidents all over again and again. Even at my day job, some events would trigger a mess in my mind. If the room was too hot, I would remember the trauma in the Narconon hot sauna. If my supervisor spoke to me rudely or cross a human rights line I thought violated, I would stand up in anger … then become dizzy — filled with anxiety. Any unexpected loud noises would freak me out until I knew what the noise was coming from.

Sleep escaped me more each night, daytime exhaustion was painful and nauseating. Depression was at my doorstep and anxiety attacks were debilitating.

A Cry for Help

Early one evening, an anxiety attack hit me hard. I had trouble breathing, was dizzy — I called 911 for help. I didn't know what else to do. An ambulance arrived and I was taken to hospital emergency. I was admitted and sedated for two days. I don't remember seeing any nurses or much about being in my hospital bed or my surroundings.

The third day, I was sitting in an office talking to a doctor. My briefcase sat beside me. I don't remember bringing it to the hospital, but I often carried it with me or had it by my side. Maybe the ambulance medics grabbed it for me or I asked them to — I don't remember, that night was a blur. The doctor asked me how I was feeling and why I called the ambulance for help.

As I was telling him about my escape from the cult of Scientology's Narconon, and some of the horrific incidents, I noticed the doctor just sitting across from me with a blank stare. He didn't understand much of what I was saying. Perhaps my words were not coming from my mouth the way my mind was trying to assemble them. I wondered if he was going to commit me to a psych ward. I stopped talking. My hand was on my briefcase.

I still thank God that I had that briefcase with me that day. It was full of documents I had taken with me from Narconon. Without having them with me in that room, who knows what course my life would have taken. I began showing the doctor these evidence documents which I was preparing for submission to government authorities, along with photos I had tucked in a side pocket of my satchel. Once the doctor saw documentary evidence of the incidents I was trying to describe at Narconon, he stopped me mid-sentence and said, "I understand now, David, and I want you to see a specialist." He immediately made a call.

Minutes later, another doctor entered the room and a few words were exchanged in French. The first doctor I saw left. Not being bi-lingual, I didn't know what was said. The doctor introduced himself and I told my story again in detail, and he diagnosed me with PTSD. He seemed genuinely concerned and phoned someone, again speaking in French. After hanging up, he assured me someone from a Crisis Center was coming to talk to me. He recommended I go for some rest and talk to staff about my distress and inability to cope very well. I agreed and waited in another room. After about an hour, a lady walked in and sat down to talk with me about my distress.

We left a short while later and drove to the outskirts of Montreal, arriving at a place that looked like a huge house from the outside. Inside was a different story — it was a crisis center for battered women, suicidal people and an office with a hot-line for people in distress. Some had been there for just two or three days, some for a week. I spent ten full days in this house, working with staff, trying to unfold my layers of confusion and anxiety. Some staff had never seen a case like mine before — someone who had been in the grip of a cult and had escaped into what seemed like a wilderness of unknowns, unable to cope in society.

Even though I was surrounded by Crisis staff I trusted, I still felt alone and being far away from home nagged at me most of the time. I did feel safer, slept better somewhat, and only had a few bad dreams that woke me up some nights.

The staff were always willing to lend an ear and listen to how I was feeling, and examined the documents and websites with me that proved what I was saying was true. An appointment was made for me with the 'Organization of the CAVAC' — a team with expertise in the areas of socio-judicial intervention and post-traumatic and continuous training to enable CAVAC staff to intervene effectively in crises. My CAVAC intervener had extensive knowledge of the judicial system, which enabled them to inform and assist me in the judicial process adequately for filing formal complaints.

On the day of my appointment, it was snowing heavily, a foot or so already piled up on the sidewalks and side streets. I followed my handwritten directions, transferring from one bus to another and somehow arriving on time. The CAVAC staff member explained what my options were. I could file a formal complaint with CCST (Quebec Workers Compensation Board) for being unable to work due to Narconon's actions *or* I could file a complaint with the Human Rights Commission, College of Physicians, and other government agencies.

The CAVAC staff member was very good, and I was out the door after my one hour visit to go back to the crisis center. The snow was thick and wet-heavy more so than when I arrived and I began trudging over to where I thought the bus stop was. After about thirty minutes, I knew I was lost — not having a clue where I was. Cold, wet and tired turned to being exhausted and frustrated — unable to decide what direction to go.

Reaching into my pocket to keep my hands warm, I found a business card. It was the card that was given to me by staff at the crisis center with their phone number on the back. I found a phone booth and called for help. "Where are you, David, can you see a street number, address or business name," asked a staff member? I gave them the name of the business I was standing beside, and within twenty minutes or so, I was in their warm car

The Road to Healing: Post-Traumatic Stress Disorder

heading back to the Center.

It hit me and tears came to my eyes. Such a simple thing to realize. I was in the care of trusted human beings. Such a contrast to my hellish treatment inside the cult of Narconon.

Following my ten day stay at the Crisis Center, I was driven to another location near Montreal.

This would be my fifth move in only a few weeks after my escape. First, I was hidden away for three days in a motel by a Federal employee, then to a house outside Montreal — followed by a three day stay in hospital which landed me in the Crisis Center, and now to another house. Within two days I found a job that hired English speaking employees as a telemarketer in a firm of three hundred in Dorval near the Montreal airport. I worked long, hard hours for a few weeks until I could afford my own apartment closer to work.

But without a doubt, I was still being followed. Montreal is huge with a population close to two million that spans over a metropolitan land area over four thousand square kilometres.

I lived in Lachine, a borough within the city of Montreal with forty-one thousand people. I lived in a rough area of town, but it was cheap and all I needed. To me, there wasn't a chance in hell that I would run into an ex-student while walking to the mall ... and the chances of running into him a second time within a two block area was not coincidence. This person would had to have known when I left my apartment and what route I would have taken in order to have met me on the sidewalk.

"Hey Dave, how are you doing, we should go for coffee at the mall someday," he said casually.

Stunned with meeting him a second time, I said, "Sure, just email me and we can meet." He never did contact me, nor did I ever see him again.

Yet I knew in my gut that he was up to no good and most likely a "Narconon Friendly" sent to spy on me. I wasn't paranoid, never have been, and I certainly was not afraid. My gut feeling was right. He was on my Facebook as a friend and when I posted something one day that was anti-Narconon, he jumped in spewing and posting pro-Narconon crap. He was one of the first people I blocked from my Facebook account.

Dante's Eighth Circle

While in the middle of these stressful moves, I met with two Quebec SQ Intelligence Agents (Sûreté du Québec) who wanted to interview me and see the documents I had from Narconon.

I was asked what I was wearing and given directions to a gas station where I was told to wait for an 'unmarked' gray van to pull up to me, then jump in the sliding side door and sit in the back. The driver pulled out of the parking lot and headed down to a restaurant and parked. We just sat there for a couple minutes with the two Agents looking around until I was told it was OK to get out of the van and follow them.

We walked into a restaurant with a few customers sitting here and there and stood near the entrance for less than a minute before one Agent said, "No, we're not going to stay here, David, we have another place not far away from here." The next place we walked into was a mediocre, run of the mill Mom and Pop restaurant with only one or two customers sitting off to the side. "Ok, this will do fine, let's sit over here, David, where it's quiet," directed the Agent.

Even though they already had a summary of facts, I once again had to start from the beginning and detail every event, handing them documents as I spoke. More than once I was told, "Slow down, David," as I was pulling papers from my briefcase and describing the horrific abuses I alleged Scientology was guilty of. We briefly discussed Scientology being a convicted criminal organization in Canada, and what they were obviously capable of doing.

They were well versed in Scientology's presence in Canada and were concerned for my safety and the safety of the patients still at Narconon. They explained that their organization had jurisdiction over all of Québec and carries out a wide variety of mandates, including international criminal investigations, protection of public figures and the National Assembly. The 'SQ' also provides support services during serious events providing specialists in various fields, including forensic identification, cyberveillance, profiling, interventions during hostage taking, and electronic surveillance. I was informed they could and would investigate my claims, but at no time would they appear in court to testify. "We will investigate and present the evidence to the appropriate authority or prosecutor," they said.

The meeting wrapped up with the agents instructing me how to avoid being followed, and if I was, how to notice a 'tail' and what to do. The intense meeting lasted close to two hours before I was driven back to a place not where I was picked up, but close to it.

I left this meeting having absolutely no idea if I'd ever see the SQ again or if they would help me win the battle I had picked with Scientology's Narconon.

What was apparent now is that I was up against a bigger, meaner monster than I initially thought. But anyone who really knew me, including some executives from Narconon, were well aware that I did not scare easily and would stand my ground if threatened.

I looked in the mirror and assured myself I would slay this monster.

Others would not suffer the way I had.

I dedicated my life to shutting down Narconon in Quebec.

My tiny bachelor apartment in Lachine was turned into my 'Office Cave' where I worked long hours into the night, tapping out submission to government agencies and filing formal complaints for investigations. Some days I would get up at 8:00 am for work at my day job, then after work, jump on a bus to arrive home by early evening to begin another grueling, long night until 3 or 4 am in the morning — scanning documents and tapping away on the keyboard.

After that first meeting with SQ Agents, I did have two more conversations with them by phone — once on Skype and the other using a pay phone. They insisted I never call them using a cell — concerned that the call would be intercepted by a cell phone scanner that could hear both sides of the call and even see text messages. What were they doing to help? Were they somehow infiltrated by Scientology? Again, I had no way of knowing who to trust.

I began to notice that I was being followed and watched when I left my apartment, and had several unannounced visits by people knocking on my door at all hours. I fought back. I set up a system that allowed me to carry 2-3 video cameras and hidden recorders. I filmed anyone I thought was tailing me. No, I wasn't scared, just being cautious and alert.

The stress of living this way was taking its toll — which is exactly what Scientology wanted. Rather than hand them any advantage, I dug in and worked harder.

Dante's Eighth Circle

My Yahoo email account was hacked, I discovered the computer I had picked up at Narconon with a police escort hand been installed with a Trojan-Horse, Worm, and Keystroke logger virus. We removed the viruses, thanks to a member from the 'Anonymous Collective' (who helped me download Anti-Malwarebytes software and boot up the old XP in 'Safe-Mode') I found the exact date my XP was accessed. Between the time that I escaped on October 28, 2009 and when I picked up my XP on November 3, 2009, someone hacked through my password and accessed my files while my computer was at Narconon Canada. Screen captures showed the exact time, date and the files that were viewed.

I was being followed into cafes and to an Interac Bank machine outside of a mall in Lachine. There was a man in a white car parked not too far from the machine — looking over at me while I was making a quick cash withdrawal. As I put the cash in my pants pocket, I reached into my top jacket pocket and took out my camera. I turned it on and ran over towards the car. The car started up and sped off fast down the length of the lot out of sight. I walked around the mall corner to my bus stop and logged onto Why We Protest — a website I visited often to see if there were any private messages for me.

I was glancing down at my cell phone and keeping an eye on my surroundings, always expecting the unexpected. Within six minutes the same man in the white car from the bank, pulled up near my bus stop. I let him see I had noticed him but he just made a right turn when the light turned green and came around for a second time — driving straight up 32nd Avenue, glancing over at me as he passed by.

Still, I was not afraid. I was more pissed off than anything, and determined to use the documents I had, to hit back as hard as I could.

When I first entered Narconon "treatment," there was a lot about Scientology I didn't know. Into the wee hours of each night, I read a lot and was learning fast. I went on social forums like *Why We Protest* (WWP), *Ex Scientologist Message Board* (ESMB) and *Reaching for the Tipping Point* (RFTTP). My impression of Scientology's leader David Miscavige quickly became: he's a person with no soul. He was described as "Tiny Fists," a violent dictator who beat his staff and locked them up for months and years in Scientology's own private prison, the "Rehabilitation Project Force" (RPF). There was a compound near the town of Hemet in Riverside County, California, unofficially nicknamed "The Hole" where senior executives have reportedly been confined for years. It has been described by ex-members as comparable to that of a North Korean death camp.

The Scientology prison compound in Hemet is ringed with high fences, topped with spikes and razor wire and monitored by motion sensors to detect anyone trying to climb out of the compound. Given slop-like food to eat, and brutal human rights abuses like being forced to crawl on their knees and stand in trash cans — confessing to things they hadn't done.

This is how Scientology treated their own.

I began to understand where Narconon's "treatment" methods came from. I had lived a nightmare eerily similar to the ones I was reading about. It was beginning to make horrible sense to me who and what I was up against.

This cult of Scientology was an evil far greater than the bit that had invaded my mind and soul while at Narconon. Their ongoing methods of intimidation and harassment were a red flag that these people were not going to stop attacking me.

I was "Fair Game" and they were the relentless hunters.

The more I worked on cases for submitting formal complaints — the flash-backs to the abusive events would stop me in my tracks. I would get lost in all the open windows on my computer, and feel confused and detached from what I was trying to do. In my mind, I was revisiting the horrific events at Narconon. Of course, I wasn't back inside the cult, but every fibre in me felt like I was ... It's a difficult feeling to explain — very ugly, evil, and dark.

At times, I felt a sense of hopelessness and despair. But the deep feeling that distressed me the most was not being able to trust people. This alone was a loneliness that's particularly distressing. I need to trust people. A cult uses methods to make you distrust anyone but them. I felt like a prisoner of war in my own mind — waking up soaking wet from horrific nightmares was disturbing.

My Guardian Angel Arrives

Rather than get overwhelmed by this huge battle I had taken on, one day I realized I needed another warrior to help me fight it.

I got in touch with Mike Kropveld, director of 'Infosect' in Montreal — a non-profit charitable organization. Mr. Kropveld referred me to Dr. Gerald Wiviott, a psychiatrist practicing at the Allan Memorial Institute. I was assured he would understand my situation and be familiar with Scientology and PTSD.

Mike Kropveld was right, Dr. Wiviott knew what I was experiencing and I began to see him once a month for a few years. He insisted that I call or email him anytime I was in distress or having an anxiety attack. We both agreed that I didn't need psychiatric medications for my PTSD, nor did I want any.

I wondered how Dr. Wiviott could comprehend how I felt inside and why the flash-backs were causing me such severe anxiety attacks. I Googled his name and learned that my doctor had once experienced similar, if not worse PTSD than I had now.

Dr. R. Gerald Wiviott was a young Medic in the Vietnam War who rose to the rank of Captain Gerald S. Wiviott, field surgeon for the 1st Bn. , 46th Infantry. He saw and experienced war in the trenches, even saving the life of a baby who wasn't breathing after a midwife delivered it. Dr. Wiviott stated: "I alternately administered aspiration and artificial respiration until the baby began to breathe on its own." After returning to the USA, Dr. Wiviott moved to Montreal — narrating his experience with the war in a book, "Hell No We Won't Go: Vietnam Draft Resisters in Canada." When Wiviott was first approached by author Alan Haig-Brown about appearing in the book, he hesitated, stating:

"I wasn't sure I wanted to think about those events again. I came to Canada to put that whole experience behind me." Wiviott says he sometimes wonders if he should have come earlier instead of serving in Vietnam. "I would have avoided some very painful things, but those events helped shape the person I am today."

I was thrilled to have a physician who knew the pain of PTSD ... he knew what I was experiencing, and I felt more relieved than I had in a very long time. Finally, here was someone I could tell absolutely everything to, be believed and not judged. Here was a doctor I could trust. And even though he had experienced the horrors of war first hand, he was still amazed at times, about what I was having to endure at the hands of Scientology and their dirty tricks, private intelligence organization, 'Office of Special Affairs'.

The Road to Healing: Post-Traumatic Stress Disorder

Of course, I thought, all psychiatrists must know about Scientology and their front group 'Citizens Commission on Human Rights' — a Scientology entity that hates psychiatrists and declared all-out war against them. "L. Ron Hubbard regarded psychiatrists as denying human spirituality and peddling fake cures. He was also convinced that psychiatrists were themselves deeply unethical individuals, committing "extortion, mayhem and murder." And Hubbard's replacement, David Miscavige, has carried forward the war against psychiatrists and the medications they prescribe. This brings us back to Narconon where these life-saving, prescribed medications are taken away, resulting in attempted suicides at their drug rehab centers, and in some cases, death to members of Scientology. In fact, according to one ex-IAS member and other source documents, if any member of Scientology is on these psych meds, they are denied auditing services.

As Dr. Wiviott learned more about Narconon and Scientology, he became quietly determined to help me heal, realizing that I was fighting a war and that I would not stop until every battle was won.

When I completed the Narconon program on May 1, 2009, I was asked by the Graduate Officer who signs off on the 'Good-To-Go' documents, "David, do you believe in reincarnation?" I replied with, "No, I do not — I have my own belief and faith in God, and I know where I'm going when I die, and it's not back here." Sometimes I wonder if the flash-backs from having PTSD will ever go away completely and I'll be normal again without having to think about it. I believe it will. I think that having a positive attitude, faith, and being around people I trust and love, makes all the difference in the world. I know I'll never forget what happened to me and others. My mind can be overwritten, just like a computer hard drive is, with new events, good experiences, and good thoughts. Indeed, it made me who I am today.

Chapter 2

Vancouver to Scientology's Narconon in Quebec

With peaks of joy and valleys of heartache, life is a roller coaster ride, the rise and fall of which defines our journey. It is both scary and exciting at the same time. —Sebastian Cole

For years I felt trapped in an underground world of prescription drug addiction, unbelievable chaos, and nightmarish thoughts. "What could I do to clean myself up and rid myself of the chains of being dragged down day in and day out?" I thought.

The daily battle within my mind far outweighed any physical pain or suffering as each day, often by the hour, I would struggle with giving in to what seemed like the easy way out. Of course, I knew that numbing my mind was only a temporary fix — an insane cycle that I knew all too well and I hated it.

At 56 years old, I felt ashamed and wanted to sink into the earth and be invisible to my family and friends — "Just leave me alone to die in peace," I thought. Living in the East End of Vancouver was a crazy life, where days and nights melted into each other — where there was no real measure of time or reality.

The turmoil in my mind was only another numbing dose away to escape, but I wanted out. This time I was more than determined. I knew it could be done if I thought about it enough and had help. I desperately craved a free and clean life but was lost in the bottles of prescriptions. Because of the extreme, high dose of 180 milligrams of prescribed methadone each day, not even the detox centers would dare admit me. First, I needed to reduce my dose down to 30-40 mg per day.

"You must wean down to about forty milligrams, David, before we can treat you," stated the intake counsellors. On top of the methadone, I was using morphine to kill my back pain and numb me. All I wanted was to get the hell off the bloody methadone. I screamed inside my mind — sometimes out loud hoping someone would shout back and answer me!

"There must be a way," I thought, and I couldn't stop searching for solutions to rid myself of this evil. I tried on my own, to reduce the dose, but the sickness that resulted took me back up to 180. To detox cold turkey from 180 mg was dangerous and unheard of, and I was desperate ... I hated being chained to a drugstore.

"Ok, I'll go for broke," I thought, "If government detox centers wouldn't accept me and help me get off Methadone, I would do it in a Vancouver hospital, whether they agreed to it or not." What happened next, I dare say some would think I was nuts, and maybe I was close to it at the time. I was at the end of my rope and very desperate. Some may have thought I should be locked up in a psych ward perhaps, but I really didn't care what people thought about me. I was going to get off Methadone come hell or high water.

What I did was so bizarre and wild, that when I think back to it, it seems like something I dreamed about or saw in a B-Movie at a cheap theatre.

When I now click my mouse on the scanned hospital records in my computer files, the reality of what happened, flashes me back to the events like it was only a few days ago.

Perhaps my daughter, Maria's words to me about being "eccentric" are truer than I know, as Webster defines: "Deviating from an established or usual pattern or style and conventional or accepted usage or conduct especially in odd or whimsical ways." What I was about to do was not only unconventional ... It was deadly.

Some say I'm "a loose cannon and beat my own drum," that I do things that many wouldn't dare try or attempt. I see myself as just someone who is tenacious and stubborn, never giving up. Many times I had gambled with my life, so why not roll the dice again ... It was a carefully, calculated risk.

Early the next morning I headed down to 'InSite' — a place I knew to be safe if an overdose occurred. The team there, led by a nurse, is available to intervene immediately and save a life if needed.

My Methadone dose that day was the norm, and hopefully it was my last.

I had a prescription of Clonidine that I knew would lower my blood pressure, and Valium would lower my heart rate. My plan was, that these two drugs, mixed with my methadone, along with a high dose of morphine would surely overdose me. I knew I would be under the watchful eyes of staff that would call an ambulance and send me off to the hospital when I collapsed.

About thirty minutes before entering 'Insite', I took an unhealthy dose of Clonidine and Valium and went in with the Clonidine hidden in one of my coat pockets — then threw the rest of the Valium away.

I didn't give much thought to the possibility of dying from this lame-brain plan I had concocted. Surely I would be saved by the nurses and medics when they arrived to reverse the drug's effects, and taken away in an ambulance.

I checked into 'Insite' that day using my Code password name "Chess-Love" — an ironic name I picked, hoping to win this real life chess game of addiction, and hopefully not fall over dead "Check-Mated." I remember sitting down at the stainless steel counter, staring in the mirror, and then I went blank.

When I woke up, I was in the cardiac ward at Vancouver General Hospital. The room seemed extremely bright as I slowly opened my eyes and looked around. I was groggy, confused and didn't know where I was.

A doctor who was standing by my bed said, "David, we almost lost you twice, your heart stopped and your blood pressure is still very low. We're not sure why your heart beat is still not back to normal." I replied, "Please don't give me any Methadone, I don't want any ever again ... But you can give me morphine or something else in small doses to relieve the withdrawal pains." The doctor agreed and when nobody was in the room, I would sneak Clonidine from my coat pocket to keep my blood pressure low so the doctor wouldn't discharge me from the hospital. As I expected, my heart rate and blood pressure remained low ... I was determined to stay in the hospital.

A few days later the doctor said he was considering a pace maker to increase my heart rate and keep it stable and that they would video image my heart to help diagnose my problem. "Sure, go ahead," I said, staring up at the ceiling wondering what would happen next. A nurse came in, wheeled me upstairs to a room, and hooked me up to a machine. I could actually see my heart and hear valves pumping blood. Although my heart rate may have been too slow for the doctor's liking, it looked fine to me ... But what did I know, maybe I'd messed something up, and I really would need a pacemaker? I really didn't care if I had a pacemaker or not — as long as I was off methadone, I would be a happy camper.

The next day, Dr. Anderson, a psychiatrist, paid me a visit. He was a nice guy and I had a gut feeling he knew what I was doing to keep my heart symptoms a mystery for as long as possible. Or, maybe the blood sample and tests returned positive for too much Clonidine in my system and he thought I was suicidal?

Thinking back to what I did, it seems unbelievable that I, or any other sane person, would do such a dangerous thing — risking death to be drug free and clean. But I felt I would be dead soon anyway, living on the streets of East End Vancouver, so I had nothing to lose by trying.

I trusted Dr. Anderson — he seemed so concerned about my condition and expressed a sincere caring. So, I told him I was taking the Clonidine that I hid in my coat on the chair. Once I explained why I had done this, he seemed to understand. In the back of my mind though, I had fears of men in white coats taking me away to a psych ward for observation. But I guess it was obvious I wasn't suicidal and only wanted to live a better life — something only a sane person wants.

The next day the Clonidine was gone from my coat pocket, but I didn't care. After being in the hospital for several days, not taking methadone, the doctors and nurses did a great job keeping me from going into severe withdrawals.

With no Clonidine, my blood pressure slowly returned to near normal and the doctor was satisfied I didn't need a pace-maker. I was in the cardiac ward for nine full days without any methadone. Finally, I was on my way to freedom!

When I was discharged, I asked the doctor if I could have a copy of my medical record, and was given a document that stated my condition as "Bradycardia." I left the hospital with a prescription of morphine and other meds in low doses and within a few days was in the Vancouver Detox Center to finish withdrawing.

While at the center, I suffered a grand mal seizure and was rushed to hospital emergency in an ambulance, unconscious. When I woke up in the hospital, I didn't know my name or where I was. It was a terrible feeling of confusion, including a severe head ache. I had been taking medication for epilepsy for many years, and I sort of knew I had a seizure. I knew these feelings of confusion and memory loss would go away soon.

After the doctor examined me, I left in a taxi back to the Vancouver Detox, with a prescription for Ativan that I filled at a pharmacy. When I arrived back at the detox, I gave the bottle to staff who continued to administer each dose as directed.

I knew there was no bloody way I could simply leave the Vancouver Detox clean and stay clean without some help. I talked to the detox counsellor and he found a three month treatment center near Vancouver for me to go to. It seemed like a great place and I felt relieved. I actually began to smile again and laugh — something I hadn't done in a long time.

I was in a good mood and happy so I called my daughter at Narconon Trois-Rivières in Quebec to tell her the good news … that I was finally off methadone and clean. She had gone to Narconon for drug treatment and after finishing the 3-4 month program, was hired on as an Ethics Officer. When I told her I was waiting to go to a treatment center in BC for three months, she asked me to "come to Narconon, it's a great treatment program." The Vancouver detox counsellor let me use the computer to Google "Narconon Trois-Rivières" to see what it was like. When I saw the advertised 70% success rate, it seemed like a dream come true. I called my daughter back and said I didn't have $23,000 to pay for Narconon — I was on Employment Insurance at $780 bi-weekly. She told me to call back the next day after she spoke to Narconon executives and the Registrar.

We hadn't seen each other for quite some time, and when I called back, she was happy to tell me that "if you agree to give Narconon your Employment Insurance income, you could do the program for half price at $11,500." I agree to the proposal and she took out a small bank loan to cover the couple thousand dollar difference. I eventually paid her back in full in monthly payments.

"It's only a three month program, Dad, and then you can go back home to

BC," she said. The Registrar sent a glowing Narconon promotional package to my counsellor, stating in the email that Narconon had a 76% success rate.

Narconon was a strange word for a treatment center that I'd never heard before. The name reminded me of the many 'Narcotics Anonymous' meetings I had gone to over the years. I really liked those meetings and what was said and learned, as well as meeting new clean and sober friends. I soon learned that 'Narconon' was the farthest thing that one could ever imagine from the other places I had ever gone to.

I wasn't looking forward to travelling on the long flight to Quebec, and was stressed and apprehensive about a drug rehab center that I knew nothing about. All this was over-shadowed by wanting to see and visit with my daughter who I had not seen in a long time.

Early the next morning, a taxi picked me up from Vancouver Detox and dropped me off at the airport. I was nervous, and still had some aches and muscle pains from methadone withdrawals. My flight wasn't for a while yet and the first place I saw in the airport was a Bar & Grill — a place I would chill at until ready to leave. I sat there sipping whiskey and taking Ativan to help keep me calm.

Not being down on the streets of the East End, I felt peaceful while sitting at the bar, but had mixed feelings. I was alone and lost in my thoughts ... "Why didn't I just stay in the Vancouver area and visit with my other two children, Jason and Maria? *Why* go all the way across Canada, when I could begin right here at home?" I mulled over these thoughts as I sucked on a piece of ice.

Finishing my drink, I let out a long sigh and headed over to wait for my flight to board. "Oh, well," I thought, "in a few more hours I'll be in Quebec — French Canada and soon see what this Narconon place is all about."

During the flight, I had a couple more drinks and some Ativan to help numb my anxiety and feelings of despair and fear. I tried to sleep, but, as usual, sore eyes stayed open and my mind wandered with numerous scenarios of what could be in store for me and what and who I was leaving behind.

Groggy and confused, I walked outside of the Montreal airport, escorted by a Narconon employee into what felt like a walk-in freezer. It reminded me of being down below in the hold of a commercial fishing boat off the west coast of Canada, while packing cod fish with ice.

When I left Vancouver it was warm enough not to wear a jacket, but this land in Quebec felt like what I imagined to be Siberia. I distinctly remember clouds of foggy, cold breath in front of me as we walked to the fancy Narconon van.

"Oh well, it's only for three months I kept reassuring myself, then I can return home." At least that's what the Narconon staff told me on the phone, including my daughter.

And ... the Narconon Registrar, Scott Burgess, claiming an incredible 76% success rate sounded promising — even though it was hard to believe.

The Narconon van driver was a friendly sort and I soon fell asleep listening to the driver's non-stop, boring chit-chat.

On Friday evening, November 28, 2008, I arrived at my daughter's apartment in Trois-Rivières. It was a medium sized apartment complex with several units rented by Narconon employees who worked at the center. I was told that Narconon didn't receive new intakes on the weekend so I would have to stay with my daughter until Monday.

Soon after I arrived, Narconon staff was dispatched to the apartment to see if I was in a sober and cooperative state. Once satisfied I was able to listen and respond, I was told to drink a solution called Cal-Mag. It was an L. Ron Hubbard concoction of calcium, magnesium and vinegar. Then, I slugged down a handful of vitamins called "drug-bombs." I was still pretty whacked out of it from drinking whiskey and popping pills on the flight, so I really didn't care, but thought, "Drub-Bombs ... The last thing I need right now is anything to do with drugs. What a dumb name for vitamins." The solution smelled sour, but I obeyed and down the hatch went a throat clogging bunch of orange-yellow pills and nasty-tasting glass of putrid vinegar and other crap like nothing I've ever tasted.

I still had the bottle of Ativan in my pocket and handed it over to my daughter, as requested. Scott instructed my daughter to keep giving the pills to me as prescribed so that I wouldn't become anxious and want to head back home. I would learn later why it was so important for me not to leave.

Perhaps I took a few too many Ativan and drinks on the flight just before landing. I was in a blubbering state of confusion, disoriented, and really didn't care much about anything — agreeing to whatever they asked of me.

As is my character and personality, I joked and laughed a lot for a while with people in the apartment that I had never met before, except for my daughter. I was asked to go lay down on a black, blown up type of air mattress that the Narconon staff would use as a kind of massage table — it was only about two feet off the floor.

Indoctrinated into Scientology

"Ok Dave, now lie on your back and relax … I'm going to give you a 'Touch Assist' — just respond "yes" when I ask you when my finger touches you," said the young man. He was a skinny kid who barely looked old enough to shave.

"What the hell is this all about," I thought, as my body sunk deep into the giant black air mattress. It was a strange place, weird practices, and people using words they made up, it seemed.

"Feel my finger," he said, as he firmly pressed into a point on my body. "Yes," I responded and then a reply of "Thank you," from the young lad.

This process of "feel my finger — yes — thank you," continued on for quite some time. I later learned, he had a fancy title of "Withdrawal Specialist." I felt no different and wondered what the hell they hoped would be the productive outcome of this nonsense on the mattress? I just laughed every time my daughter's black cat jumped up onto me.

After a short break, another hand full of vitamins, I sunk into the living room sofa hoping to have a nap. But, no rest yet — Narconon had more so-called therapy routines lined up for me.

My daughter sat across from me in the living room and asked me to do what she called a simple training routine. Later, I would learn that these 'touch assists' and other routines, were to keep me in what Scientology calls 'Present Time'. Apparently, thinking back over ones' past is not healthy according to L. Ron Hubbard. The Narconon staff looked upon Hubbard as some kind of god or genius, and worshipped his words as god-like. They believed that Hubbard's words were the solution to all of mankind's mental health problems, and would clear the planet of crime, drugs, and psychiatrists.

"Ok dad, just sit there still and stare at my face without moving," she said with a smile. "No problem," — I hadn't seen my daughter for a long time, so this was nice and I smiled back. First I had to sit with my eyes closed for several minutes, then with eyes open.

The young lad who did the 'touch assist' said laughing, "Wow, Dave can do this well — probably because he's on Ativan." Staring at my daughter's face for so long, had me seeing double and pieces of her face features melting off to the sides. "What a trip," I thought!

Then we started what someone called "Light Objectives" — another strange new experience that made me even more tired, and wondering "what the hell have I landed myself into now?" I was commanded to: "Look around the room and find something that is green" — then "look around the room and find something that is blue," and on and on until I was frustrated and exhausted. It was so tiring that I don't even remember who was giving the commands.

Finally, I lay down on the couch and the others went off to bed. A while later, my daughter came into the living room to see if I was OK, and I told her I was definitely NOT OK and couldn't fall sleep!

The next morning after a rough night, I was taken to the mall to buy a warm jacket and other cloths I would need, including a wool toque to keep my ears from freezing. It was extreme cold outside with snow piled high.

Saturday and Sunday at the apartment was a nightmare. The Ativan bottle was almost empty. I was feeling withdrawals from the pills … and even more so from my five years of taking methadone every day. Nine days in the hospital and five days in Vancouver detox was not quite enough time to feel well again and back to normal.

Sleep was impossible, confusion and mental torment was a constant. I feared having another seizure like I had in Vancouver Detox, and I knew well, that another seizure was only a matter of time if I didn't see a doctor for my anti-seizure medication, Dilantin.

I remembered seeing people in the apartment drinking beer and wine. It seemed strange to see the fridge shelves lined with alcohol in an apartment where people lived, just out of the Narconon drug rehab.

But I needed something to help me sleep, and woke my daughter up, asking for a glass of wine. She said, "Ok," but insisted that I not tell anyone for fear of her being in trouble. She went over to the counter and returned with a glass of wine and an Ativan. I didn't give it too much thought, but again wondered, "Why does my daughter, after completing the Narconon program, have wine in her apartment?" Knowing some of her history, I was pretty sure the alcohol was not just for guests?

Still, sleep was difficult... Confusion and mental torment was a constant, and I knew well, the nightmare ahead. A few gulps of wine and minutes later I was sound asleep in pleasant dream-land.

Perhaps it was a good thing that I didn't have my wits about me when I awoke the next morning? Anyone in their right mind would have asked a ton of questions. Like, what the hell was all this strange staring, touchy-feel-my-finger, and looking around a room for colours was all about. But most people arriving for treatment at a drug rehab, including me, really don't care about much, we just want to get it over with and return home as soon as possible.

"Let's just get on with it, and get the hell out of here," was all that mattered to me.

Chapter 3
Painful Beginnings in the Cult Compound

> STOP! *You are not permitted to talk about Scientology while in the Narconon program.*

Monday morning, December 1, 2008, I arrived at the Narconon Trois-Rivières rehab center. The buildings were old, run-down, and resembled a massive homeless shelter or photos I'd seen of old, closed down prisons. It was nothing like any other drug rehab treatment center I had ever seen.

Staff members were walking around with walkie-talkies counting people, and even though they were patients suffering from a severe illness, they were referred to as "students." It was a very strange place that didn't fit into any of my past memories of anything.

When I noticed a huge Catholic Crucifix outside the window near some trees, I was told the complex used to be a convent. Now I understood why the buildings were so old and run down and seemed like an institution of sorts.

"A few Nuns still live here over at the far building, but we seldom see them," said one of the Narconon staff.

I sat down in a room that looked like a dining room of an old home or a shabby conference room in a real estate office. Minutes later, I was greeted by the registrar, Scott, a tiny shell of a man. He was hardly the person I had imagined while I was speaking to him on the phone in Vancouver. He sat down beside me and laid out some documents, which he had wanted me to read and sign.

"Read them?" I asked, "Are you kidding me!" I could barely sit up straight in the chair. My rational thinking was non-existent, to say the least. I grabbed the documents, ran my finger down the pages, and scribbled my name on the bottom line. I had no clue what I had signed and really didn't care. I just wanted to lie down and rest.

After I signed, a smirk widened on his skinny, unshaven little face as he stood up and beckoned to John (not real name), the scruffy looking senior 'Ethics Officer' I had met at my daughter's apartment. John was her boyfriend, who lived in the same apartment complex where I had been during the weekend.

After seeing how he behaved in the apartment over the weekend, I had little respect for this so-called Ethics Officer. My first impression of him remains, namely that, he was (and still is) a creepy crawler who could not be trusted or respected.

John took me across the parking lot over to the withdrawal unit. I put my bag of clothes and personal belongings on the table. After a quick search, I was escorted into what looked like a tiny hospital clinic with two massage tables in the middle of the hallway.

I had forgotten about my black air mattress 'touchy-touchy' experience until I heard someone say, "Feel my finger" over and over again. When the student mumbled "YES", the staff member would respond with rotating relies of "excellent" — "awesome" and "very good"... like some kind of robot implanted with a memory chip. It was eerie and strange listening to it.

After a quick shower I was off to my new tiny bedroom that had two beds squeezed in on each side of the room.

The Interrogations Begin

Moments later a staff person appeared with the memorable drug bombs, Cal-Mag and a clip board with pen in hand.

"Now what," I thought as I saw the clip board and sat up to gag down the concoction.

"I need to ask you some questions about your drug use history," said Jessica (not real name), a tall, thin lady with dark hair. She was very nice

Painful Beginnings in the Cult Compound

and I said "sure, no problem, let's do it." She called herself a 'Withdrawal Specialist' and began to probe for answers. After a couple hours of interrogations, she said, "David, I give up, you are getting too angry and frustrated" and stopped the interview.

I was in no mood to answer her questions about my past years of drug use, never mind her insisting I confess to decades back. I really couldn't remember or care, and her persistence was seriously pissing me off. "To hell with them," I thought, and lay back down.

The symptoms of Ativan and residual Methadone withdrawal, with bone aching pain, were beginning to consume my thoughts. Disoriented, I just thought of my children back home, and being with them in British Columbia.

Here I was, stuck thousands of miles from home in what seemed like a circus of confusion and very strange people doing weird things to so-called students.

"Did I make a big mistake coming here ... Where is the doctor or nurse," I thought. The uneasy feeling was overwhelming and I was distressed to my limit.

The next morning, my daughter appeared in my room, and sat on the bed across from me with the familiar clipboard in hand.

The withdrawal specialist Jessica, had quite the time with me the previous day trying to get coherent medical information so they must have thought my daughter would have better luck. But, I was in no mood to answer questions of any sort and said: "I can't do this here, I'm going back home as soon as possible."

"Just one more day, Dad — just stay another day," she replied. "C'mon Dad, just answer a few more questions for your file and we're done." After a moan, I spewed out a few more answers and she left.

Unbeknown to me at the time, "confidential" was a mere misinterpretation on my part as I would learn in the near future.

The next day a young lad was booked into my bedroom in a bed across from me. He was a funny guy and this was his second time at Narconon for what they called a "REPAIR." My roommate seemed like an intelligent sort and I liked him.

He said to me, "Dave, I was so messed up the day Narconon called that when I looked at my call display I thought it said the Narc Police were calling." He said he was in a state of mental psychosis from using too much cocaine and was paranoid as hell. We both laughed but it wasn't funny, the chuckle was short-lived.

I grabbed my cigarettes and went out to the deck with my new roommate at the end of the withdrawal unit. It was freezing cold and a couple of puffs were enough for me and back to my room I went.

Moments later a staff member called me into the kitchen area where there was a tiny desk at one end, a small kitchen counter with cupboards and a small table in the center. The area was much smaller than in most homes and over cramped with the seven students that were there.

I sat in a chair facing the staff member … It was the dreaded light objectives I had experience at the apartment. Commands of "look around the room and find something that is this color or that color" soon had me in a dizzy pain. I just wanted to be left alone so I could curl up in bed in a fatal position. When I pulled my knees up to my chest, my back pain wasn't as bad.

But as soon as the light objectives were finished I was told to get up on the massage table for a "nerve assist." This was another process where their hands drag down your back, arms and legs. This actually felt good and I didn't have to respond with "yes." A few times I drifted off into a sleep for a few minutes.

An old guy was giving me an assist one day and I asked what this was supposed to do? "To calm the nerves and relax muscles," he replied.

The only thing that seemed to somewhat relieve my muscle aching pains, was taking hot Epsom salt baths often in a small bathtub.

I was in the withdrawal unit for about 10-12 days, and the average time for other students was from 3-6 days, so I saw many come and go. It was co-ed rehab with men and women. Some coming off opiates were sick as dogs and couldn't keep down food, puking on the floors — not a pretty sight or smell in such small confines.

Even worse, were the effects from swallowing toxic doses of vitamins every few hours. There were so many pills in a single dose that I had to split them into two gulps. Every student had severe diarrhoea and with only one tiny bathroom for seven students and staff, it was a smelly, disgusting mess. Most students suffered with ass-burning diarrhoea for about two months until they completed the Narconon sauna part of the program. And our urine was a bright, almost fluorescent yellow-green colour.

A group of us were sitting around one day and my roommate was telling us stories of his first time through the program. "This place is run by Scientology you know and that's what they will teach you here," he said.

As soon as Jessica, the Withdrawal Specialist, overheard him talking to us about the Narconon program being Scientology, she interrupted the conversation and said loudly: "STOP — you are not permitted to talk about Scientology while in the Narconon program." I was stunned and wondered why the hell not — this is Canada, a land of free speech, freedom of expression, and freedom of religion. Even if it was Scientology, I and probably most others, didn't have a clue what the hell it was anyway, so what's the big deal, I thought?

Later that afternoon, I approached a staff member on the night shift and asked why we couldn't discuss Scientology?

He said, "David, if one of the students calls home when they are out of withdrawal and mentions to their parents or sponsor that Scientology is discussed here, they may pull the student out of the program and place them somewhere else."

I still didn't know anything about Scientology, what it was, and couldn't understand what he was talking about. His explanation didn't make any sense to me whatsoever, but I let it go and focussed on dealing with me, and how I was going to deal with and handle all this.

I was in no mood to argue so I just went to my room again and curled up in a ball. They say your sins shall find you out and they sure as hell did here in Québec. What an unexpected, bloody nightmare.

I woke up the next day with a screaming headache, disoriented, and didn't know my name or where I was. I lay in bed staring at the ceiling, cold and scared — my ears ringing. Within a few minutes I realized what had happened. I knew I had another grand mal seizure while here in the withdrawal unit.

"Why wasn't I in the hospital," I thought? I got out of bed and carefully walked into the kitchen where a staff member was sitting at the desk. I told him what happened and he replied that I was probably only dreaming. "This was no bloody dream — I had a seizure — "I know exactly how they feel, do you?" I replied in anger.

I explained to him that I had a seizure in the Vancouver Detox before coming here and they rushed me to emergency in an ambulance to treat and care for me. "This is serious, I've had many falls on hard floors — look at all the scars under my chin. These are from seizures," I said.

"Do you have any idea what it feels like to not know your name or who you are or where you are," I explained. I was furious when the so-called Withdrawal Specialist insisted I didn't have a seizure. It was like talking to somebody who couldn't hear me, didn't understand what I was saying, or simply didn't care what I was saying!

"Where is the doctor and nurses — when will I see one?" I asked.

"students see the doctor in Montreal on Wednesdays only and we will take you there," he replied.

"Are you kidding me? That's tomorrow and I'm too sick to be able to travel in a van for the three hours round trip," I said. He could see I was not a happy camper.

He then took my pulse and blood pressure and said I would be fine — "not to worry." My headache was going away and my thinking was clearing up some, so off to lie down and think about what happened. I was so upset and angry, but kept it inside for the time being.

Wednesday morning arrived and a staff member called over to the main building to say I was still too sick to make the trip to see Dr. Labonte in Montreal.

With plenty of doctors in Trois-Rivières, it seemed strange and ridiculous to have to travel all the way to Montreal. "Maybe he's some kind of addiction specialist," I pondered. Little did I know that he was a member of the Church of Scientology and promoted their program at every turn.

The next Wednesday rolled around and I was off to Montreal with a few other students in the Narconon van. For me, the trip was the longest trip ever — one that I wished I could erase from memory.

A Quack Doctor and the Narconon Charlatans

Finally it was my turn to leave the waiting room and see the doctor — and what a crazy visit it was. After I explained about my seizures, four back surgeries, and liver scarring, he lifted a huge book onto his desk.

"I think we can handle your issues with a vitamin regime," he said, trying to reassure me.

I told him: "Hey, no bloody way I'm not taking Dilantin, my anti-seizure medication that has been prescribed to me for years — no bloody way!" He seemed frustrated with my attitude, and his demeanour changed dramatically to one of disgust and uncaring.

"What kind of doctor-patient relationship was this," I thought, but little did I know that his relationship to the cult was far more important than caring for the health and welfare of the ill.

Reluctantly, he agreed and said: "Alright, fine, I'll continue with it." After my bewildering experience with Dr. Pierre Labonte, I was back in the withdrawal unit for a couple more days. To be certain I was in a "cooperative" state and demeanour, I had to do the TR staring session for fifteen minutes before I would be released out of withdrawal and in a dorm room with the other students.

The timer was gradually moved up from six to fifteen minutes eyes closed, then open. Once I received a pass and OK from the staff, I was out.

"Yahoo, I'm free!" I thought.

Not once, in my eleven months at Narconon as a patient or on staff, did I ever see any doctor visit the center ... Not once! Many of the Narconon staff think or pretend they are trained addiction specialists, but in fact are just dangerous Charlatans — in some cases, practicing medicine without a license.

Narconon likes to boast that they use no medications to help addicts withdraw from drugs, but this dangerous dogma is indeed a risk to health, if not deadly. One middle aged man was rushed to hospital emergency by ambulance while he was in the withdrawal unit being treated for severe alcoholism. Alcohol withdrawal can be a dangerous process without the appropriate medication, such as Phenobarbital or other anti-seizure medication. Many severe alcoholics are monitored closely in a hospital setting during severe withdrawals. Narconon was not qualified, nor did it have medical staff to safeguard health and safety.

I think the infamous L. Ron Hubbard had a complete misconception of what drug addiction is. The stigma of a drug addict hiding in back alleys, robbing the elderly, and the most despised in society, is simply not the case.

In fact, at Narconon, one might be surprised at who the patients were and where they came from. Of course some were dysfunctional and unable to be productive members of society due to their addiction, but many were quite productive, well educated, and owned and operated successful businesses.

And even more importantly, they had family and loved ones waiting for them to return home safe and well ... Not pay $23,000 to be treated by unqualified quacks using pseudoscience, and relapsing shortly after returning home.

Chapter 4
A Peek into Hell: the Stairway to Nightmares

Scientology is worse than many think and their Narconon drug rehabs are dangerous and deadly above what most could ever imagine.

    I can be a hard-nosed, tough act when I see vulnerable people being abused or exploited for the almighty buck. I'll say and do whatever it takes to help those less fortunate or unable to help themselves. But there is another side to my personality and character that I live in most often — that of empathy and compassion... "Do unto others as you would have them do unto you." I think I was born with a gift that I carry with me most days that allows me to see and feel other's pain and suffering. Sometimes it's a good thing to have, other times I wish it were not there, but it is. And now, here I was, in a place where chaos was the norm at times... A place where so many people were all over the spectrum of present pain and trauma from past to present.

    The stairway up to the men's dorm was filthy — floor tiles on the steps worn through the old patterns and lifting up at the corners. There was a young guy with a six foot long, steel 'chisel-spade' type tool, digging up the flooring to replace with something new. I was told he had relapsed and returned to do the Narconon program again, paying for it in exchange for work projects.

    Once I reached the second floor, I stood in the middle of two long wings with another set of stairs that went down to the security office door to the right and exit door straight ahead to the walkway that led over to the main building.

They were small, cinder-brick rooms, with a small sink and no bathroom — communal washrooms and showers were down the hall. My room had a set of wooden bunk beds, with a small window facing off into the woods and a sand volley-ball court nearby.

I settled into my new room quickly, hanging a few clothes in the tiny closet and filling one drawer in the antique dresser. My daughter had dropped off a new diary book while I was in the withdrawal unit, so I flopped down on the bottom bunk and began writing.

I soon closed my eyes and drifted off into a blessed sleep — one of very few I would have without horrific nightmares.

A few days after I was in my dorm room, another student was bunked in on the top bunk … But not for long.

I woke up early one morning and wondered where he was? He was gone!

As I opened my bedroom door to go down to the bathroom, there he was sleeping in the hallway by the wall. "Now what the hell is he doing out here on the hard floor," I thought. I just tip-toed past him, shaking my head and did my thing.

Once he was awake I asked him why he slept out on the hard, hallway floor.

He said "David, you are the loudest sleeper I have ever heard. You snore and talk loud in your sleep! I couldn't sleep you were moving around so loud." I apologized and he was assigned a new room, leaving me to have my own private room for the duration. Security staff did room checks every so often and told me they thought I was talking to someone in my room at night.

There were few nights that I didn't have nightmares. I thought maybe it was because I was writing about all the crazy shit that happened at Narconon each day. They were disturbing, weird and scary dreams that I hated having. I would wake up often — finding myself soaked in cold sweat.

But I was determined to write about all the events of every day … "Maybe I'll write a book about this one day, and this place has a lot to tell," I thought. It was like living in a temple of evil secrecy, hate, and fear. Something about this place was definitely different.

A Peek into Hell: the Stairway to Nightmares

I had, and still do have, a strong Christian faith and beliefs and before flying to Narconon I asked them on the phone if Narconon would conflict with my beliefs. They replied, "No, absolutely not David, Narconon is not a religious drug rehab." But every day I was there, I could feel that something wasn't right — a creepy, chilling feeling inside. I just couldn't put my finger on what it was. I had no knowledge about Narconon or Scientology. I had heard the 'Hubbard' name before, but never read anything about him or Scientology.

Every spare minute I had alone, I diarized notes and hid disposable cameras and photos that new graduates gave me before they left.

My room was searched often, and the only documents I left in view were those I was sure the staff would probably read.

I would place them meticulously on my tiny two foot square table, and using a piece of string, I measured the precise distance from one corner of the stacked papers to my bedpost. When I would return after lunch or in the evening, I would measure again, noting that my pages had been moved. Sometimes, they were one or two inches from where I had placed them.

The important diarized notes were stowed away in a safe place that I only went to when absolutely necessary to hide more documents. I knew that if discovered, my writings would land me in huge trouble or have me kicked out, embarrassing and making my daughter very angry.

I didn't have much paper so I grabbed meal voting sheets and napkins to write on. While sitting in the dining room there was no shortage of what to write about. Sometimes I would get bored and just write self-esteem building poems for students having troubles. But most of my writing I kept secret and hidden.

There were about 80 students, and as many staff when I was there at the beginning, and the dorms were crowded and noisy with gatherings in the TV room and bedrooms. Many of us would walk to the main building across the parking lot and hang around the large dining room after classes and on Sundays.

Instead of having paid staff members clean the dorms, course rooms, and dining room, students were forced to work each and every day, including cleaning bathrooms, toilettes and mopping hallway floors. A staff member would simply inspect the cleanliness and report to the ethics officer any job that wasn't done to perfection. Anyone who didn't perform as commanded, was interviewed, interrogated and put through the dreaded ethics cycle. Fear of this interrogation process was apparent to those who had experienced such demoralizing questions. To some, it seemed more like a military prison camp than a drug rehab center.

After paying $23,000 to Narconon, the fact of being forced into manual labour to help run the operation of the center, seemed ludicrous to many.

And when a staff member quit because they were not paid, students took their place and slaved doing dishes or kitchen work with no remuneration whatsoever. Many times, not even a thank you or smile from executives.

One day after lunch and after a phone call to my wife back home in western Canada, I was called up to an executive office. After I sat down in her large office across from her, she said, "David, you don't know why you're here in my office, do you?"

"No I don't, why am I here," I replied?

"David, someone overheard you saying that Narconon is just a money grab," she said with a stern face.

"No I didn't," I replied, shaking my head. "I was just telling the person beside me what my wife in B. C. said to me on the phone at lunch time, that's all." The executive went on to explain how Narconon had helped so many people and that it was a non-profit organization and definitely not a "money grab." After I was dismissed, I went back to my room for a few minutes before more afternoon work in the course rooms. I couldn't believe that I was being told what I could and couldn't talk about. The executive was a strange lady, with a pasted on, fake smile — not the happiest sort. I was told later that she was one of the Narconon executives and married to the executive director, Marc Bernard. Both were Scientologists, and working there together with their combined income, earned a handsome sum.

Tarnishing Narconon's Reputation

I soon learned that anything that happened at Narconon which could tarnish Narconon's reputation was handled internally within the Scientology group of executives, and swept under the carpet. Junior staff was forbidden to discuss any abusive events or incidents of human rights abuse and health risks to students.

A Peek into Hell: the Stairway to Nightmares

Even my own daughter did not confide with me about a gun being at the staff apartment complex and an ex-Narconon student shooting himself dead. Later, after my daughter left in the middle of the night, and I escaped, I received a few emails, informing me about a death that shocked me.

Email from daughter:

"He graduated before you got there in October and killed himself a month after you were there in Jan. I never told you because you were still in WD [withdrawal] and it was hard on me ... he had been through Narconon at least three times ... Janice [not real name] threw it [gun] over the balcony to him one night ... " The young man took the gun to Ontario and shot himself dead.

When I read the emails I was stunned with the thought that guns were at the Narconon staff complex where my daughter lived. And when I 'time-lined' the tragic suicide, I wasn't in WD as my daughter wrote — it was January 1st when he shot himself and I was already in the dreadful dorms.

So, while I was bunked in these human warehouse type dooms, parties were ongoing at the Narconon apartment complex down the road. In fact, deadly parties! Not just parties with all the alcohol I had seen when I arrived, but also cocaine ... And who knows what else.

Prior to pulling the trigger and taking his own life, this now deceased young man, had been through the Narconon Trois-Rivières treatment center multiple times with no success. It was a horrific event that stirred many emotions and left a young child with no father.

After hearing the story from my daughter and the dead man's girlfriend, I wondered how such a horrific event could happen. With professional medical care and a qualified therapist, he certainly would have increased his chances of survival.

After escaping Narconon, I received numerous Facebook messages from the deceased young man's girlfriend, an ex-Narconon staff member. She had a baby with the young ex-Narconon student and confirmed what my daughter wrote to me about the death.

Dante's Eighth Circle

Messages to Me from a Young Mom

Even though leaving the center was probably one of the best decisions I have made in my life, I just was glad I was out of there. I found a new job and realized what a real work place is. No backstabbing, arguing all the time, writing other people up, and games — well you know it. I was talking to my new boss wondering why I stayed there so long. Looking back, I can't understand. It was for the students obviously, but still something was wrong.

When Johnny[1] died, I blamed the drug. He did many rehabs including 12 steps and he really believed NN was the answer. Before he went back to the center last time, he tried to commit suicide. I called the cops on him. He ended up in psychiatry. Then he was released to a homeless shelter because I did not take him back. He absolutely wanted to get back to the center. I tried to tell him that any rehab would help, he could maybe try something else, but he really wanted to go to NN and he went for free.

I was thankful because he believed in it and he was safe. Then, I knew exactly when he relapsed. Called him at lunch and he did not answer — never heard from him personally ever again. I heard he was living at Kyle's but I did not even bother to go kick the shit out of them. I just had enough. Then I heard one morning at the tech meeting from John (I think) that they called the cops on him the night before because of a gun. Then my brother called to say the cops went to his workplace with Johnny's picture looking for him stating he was dangerous and armed. I emailed his ex-wife to let her know what was up to in case he tried to get in touch with her. He did and I knew he was in Ontario. Didn't know he still had the gun and then the rest is history. I personally never talked about it at work because I had to be strong for me and my son and if I talked about it I would cry. I started to stop believing in the program, but wanted to fight addiction so much. Anyways it caught up with me. When I left I was twenty-seven and felt like forty years old.

So, this vulnerable young man was known by Narconon staff executives

---

[1] Name of deceased changed to "Johnny" in consideration of innocent child, and name of mother changed to Melody.

to be suicidal and in fact attempted to take his own life on an earlier occasion before he went back to the center the last time, and tried to commit suicide.

On April 18, 2012, Le Nouvelliste newspaper confirmed more unconscionable Narconon practices of admitting patients with suicidal tendencies and "serious problems of a psychiatric nature."

> Sylvain Bérard, the Ethics Officer, said that Narconon had already been experiencing financial problems for some time, to such an extent that, in recent months, the organization had even been admitting clients with more serious problems of a psychiatric nature.
>
> Some of these cases weren't admissible to the program because it requires cutting off their medication. But the administration chose to keep them anyway. There were several instances of attempted suicide during the past few months. By law, immediate medical assistance should have been provided, but management decided to keep these persons without calling for an ambulance," says the former employee.
>
> His colleague, Julie Ann Pagé remembers a female resident who, less than ten days earlier, made at least two suicide attempts in one day, but she was not referred to a hospital. Ms. Pagé says that incidents like this were blamed on the employees for supposedly "not delivering enough.
>
> We had no right to have a personal opinion. The only thing that mattered was their teaching of Scientology. Don't do to others what you wouldn't want them to do to you. This was one of their internal rules, but they themselves don't apply it. They have no respect for us or for the residents," says Sylvie Houde.
>
> We're playing with people's lives," adds Julie Ann Pagé."

There was no student aftercare program in place — at least not one that was based on therapeutic science. If a patient is having troubles or relapsed, they are instructed to apply some of the Scientology Training Routines, policies and doctrines they learned and were subject to while in the program.

Of course, as usual, all these horrific events are hushed up by executives. Even with my dorm wing nearly full to capacity with students at various stages of the program, I heard nothing about the 'death by gun' until after

Dante's Eighth Circle

I escaped.

Chapter 5

A Cult of Paranoia

If they can get you asking the wrong questions, they don't have to worry about answers. —Thomas Pynchon

Before I could start the Narconon program, I met in the office with the paranoid senior Ethic's Officer John, who fired a barrage of questions at me. He seemed like he enjoyed his staff position of playing interrogator, but his demeanour was laughable as he sat back in his office chair grinning. He didn't seem like, or talk like 'the sharpest pencil in the box' of the Narconon minions. He acted like a hung-over drunk at a circus event.

"David, are you here 'under-cover' as a journalist or government agent?" he asked.

I laughed out loud, thinking he was kidding — but apparently not. If I had planned to be undercover to help a journalist or the government with intelligence that they could use, I sure as hell would not tip my hand to this guy or anyone else while I was there.

"No, today I'm not — what kind of crazy question is that?" I asked.

He looked at me with a smirk: "I have to ask, it's my job," he said.

I knew who this John guy was. He was at my daughter's, apartment when I arrived, and had a few too many drinks under his belt. He was saying disgusting things and laughing. My respect for this pompous ass dropped below zero when he said, "Do you know what would look good on you?" Without waiting for an answer, John replied, "ME!" Then he staggered over to the fridge to grab another beer.

Dante's Eighth Circle

And now, this glossy-eyed dude is asking me stupid questions after binge-drinking the night before? I didn't know at the time, but it was far more than just drinking. He had relapsed back into his drug of choice, and was prancing around as the Senior Ethics Officer. Here he was playing the role of Narconon Cop, interrogating students for minor infractions, all while he himself, was committing criminal offences.

After he went over the basic student rules and schedules, I was led across the hall to Dina's 'Qual Office' where I was handed tests to complete. I then sat in a quiet, small room at the end of the hallway to answer questions on their bogus "IQ" and "Personality" tests.

The Qualifications (Qual) is a division in Narconon where the student is examined and may receive either *cramming* (special assistance) or be awarded certificates for completions. It's also where students are required to write "success stories" at each step of the program.

The personality test was two hundred questions of absolute bloody nonsense of twisted, ridiculous mind benders. TWO HUNDRED! After turning in my answers to Dina, I was called into her office to review my results. Without any explanation, she said in a matter of fact tone, "Don't worry David, this graph will improve as you go through the Narconon program and your personality score will be higher."

"Improve what?" I thought.

The "IQ Test" was much shorter. I finished a couple minutes before my time was up and handed it in.

What I didn't know is that I would have to do these tests two more times while there — once after the sauna program and again after I completed the entire program.

"Now you can begin the Narconon Book 1," Dina said as I walked out the door.

I thought to myself, "Next time I'll answer the personality test questions how I *think* they want them answered. That'll shut 'em up, eh?" Of course, I felt a hell of a lot healthier, both physically and mentally, after being clean for a month, but I knew with certainty, that Narconon didn't have anything to do with me feeling better. The program hadn't provided any treatment or professional therapy whatsoever. I probably could have gone on a long

A Cult of Paranoia

camping trip and felt much better than I did after having had my mind invaded and twisted by this cult of chaos.

Narconon had *no* doctors or nurses. Incredibly, students didn't have scheduled visits with counsellors nor were there group meetings to discuss their addiction issues. There was not one medically qualified staff member the entire time I was there, either as a "student" or as a staff member.

The cult saves money, training students to indoctrinate each other. Scientology's Narconon program is designed so that each student pairs up with another student called their "Twin" and the two remain together for the entire program. This saves Narconon huge sums by not providing qualified therapists or councillors. The con of all cons! I think one TV reporter nailed it when referring to the proposed Narconon in Frederick, Maryland, mispronouncing the name, calling it, "NarcaCON." Some Twins graduate close to the same day, and others, like me, were assigned to an 'extended' program. My extension only lasted a few days of which two full days were sessions sitting in front of Scientologists.

I was already being groomed to be recruited as a Narconon staff member. My case supervisor, Marc Bernard, called to me from the dining room sundeck one afternoon. "David, we are going to turn the marrow in your back into solid bone!" Narconon executives knew I could stand up to them and hold my ground in any conversation or dispute, so they wanted to train me to be one of their media handlers by stripping away my personality and emotions.

When one of the Twins gets into trouble and is put through an Ethics Cycle, it often resulted in forced manual labour or some other program delay. Their Twin's treatment program is also stopped. This was so unfair and didn't make sense, but not much else did either.

Many students, myself included, just want to finish as soon as possible and go home. A phrase used often by students was, "I'm being file fucked," which meant their student case file was put away and their program stoppped, for whatever reason staff felt like at the time.

My Twin was a great young lad and we got along well for 95% of the time. But nearing the end, especially when doing Narconon's *Objectives Book*, we did have our times of disagreements.

Chapter 6

First Day in the Devil's Den of Hell

It was so loud and shocking that I couldn't believe what just happened. It was the craziest, bat-shit Cuckoo's Nest thing I had ever heard!

Walking down the old stairs into what used to be a Catholic chapel was an experience that still causes sleepless nights and nightmares. There were two lines of chairs set facing each other and a few other chairs set up in pairs here and there.

My Twin and I were told to get our case of Narconon books from the course room closet and take out Book 1. After we put our names on the outside of all eight books, we put the heavy case back, and then saw the course room supervisor with Book 1, *Theraputic Training Routines (TRs)*, in hand. We were told to put the book over on the shelf beside the stack of ashtrays.

Then, we begin doing the dreaded TRs — sitting across from each other, staring towards the other with our eyes closed. I was tired, but thought, "Oh, this isn't so bad — I'll just close my eyes and drift off into a dream or think about being back home." The guy sitting next to me was kind of smiling and his head was moving slightly to what seemed like the beat of music. He wasn't moving enough to attract attention from the supervisor and I thought he was just singing songs in his head to pass time. But that wasn't the case.

It was still winter in Quebec and very cold, so the guy was wearing a toque pulled down over his ears in the course room.

I laughed my ass off when he later showed me his IPod and the earphones that his toque covered. He was listening to music while doing his TRs!

I didn't have an IPod yet or I probably would have done the same thing.

Then, just as I was half conscious, daydreaming about walking along a beach back home, I heard a blood-curdling scream: "ASHTRAY STAND UP — THANK YOU — SIT DOWN ON THAT CHAIR — THANK YOU!!!" And this was loud — as loud as one can yell or scream.

It was so loud and shocking that I couldn't believe what just happened. It was the craziest, bat-shit thing I had ever heard! They kept doing it over and over again.

Over in the chapel room beside us, I could hear commands: "You, look at that wall — You walk over to that wall" and "touch that wall — stop it from going away." Then I overheard the real winner that would eventually get me in a shit heap of distress and trouble: "Did 'YOU' keep it from going away?"

"It's a solid bloody wall, with no will to walk away! So how is a student stopping this perfectly still wall from walking away," I thought. It sounded dumber than dumb.

"What color is the bottle — how much does it weigh — what's its temperature," I could hear coming off to the side of us in a small alcove area.

A few feet away from me in the same room, a student bullbaiting their Twin was another shocking thing to watch and hear. By now, we had finished our TRs with eyes closed and could see all that was happening ... We were doing TRs with our eyes open.

In the bull baiting exercise, one Twin sits absolutely frozen still while the other does everything possible to make them smile, move or flinch without touching them. Touching would come later.

"Listen you disgusting whore, your children hate you, your boyfriend is sleeping around, and you're parents have disowned you," were just a sample of verbal assaults. It was disgusting to hear and I felt sorry for the person on the receiving end of the insults and degradation.

My Twin and I had to read L. Ron Hubbard's absurd writings in Book 1 and use the check sheet to tick off each section we finished.

At one point during the afternoon, I thought to myself: "Have I lost it? Is this real or a bad dream — or have I really blown it this time and my daughter has committed me to a nut house?" I could only compare, at that time, that the whacko craziness in these rooms were something far more insane than the Jack Nicholson movie "One Flew over the Cuckoo's Nest."

"What the hell does this have to do with any kind of addiction treatment," I mumbled on my way out for supper.

I was the oldest student there at fifty-six, and older than most of the staff, so I had experienced a lot of 'off the wall' things, but never like this. Something didn't feel right at Narconon about this house of quacks, and I often shook my head in disbelief.

"What were they not telling me? Why did I feel such uneasiness? What is wrong with me," I often wondered.

Chapter 7

A Military Compound of Surveillance and Suffering

> *There is the solitude of suffering, when you go through darkness that is lonely, intense, and terrible. Words become powerless to express your pain; what others hear from your words is so distant and different from what you are actually suffering.* —John O'Donohue

I kept on writing diarized notes of the craziness. Just when I thought I had seen it all, another event would stagger my mind. I guess I must have viewed each event by itself and not put them together — seeing only the puzzle pieces and not the full picture of horrors.

I was always interested in people — about who they were and what made them tick, and at Narconon, there were volumes of interesting souls — staff and students.

Whenever I was out on the dining room sundeck, I could see people mingling and interacting with each other. I also enjoyed sitting on the deck and having long chats with the students. Inside the dining room, people were snacking and sitting around playing games and such.

Getting a straight answer, or any answer at all from most staff, was next to impossible. The dumbest things spewed from their mouths. It was like they were holding close, scary secrets. I could see the fear and uneasiness on their faces and in their cautious, whispering demeanour.

Watching the security guards and student control staff walking around with walkie-talkies and clip boards, reminded me of an old black and white prison movie that I couldn't get the drift of.

Every twenty minutes or so, they would walk around counting us and noting on the clip board paper where we were and who we were with.

They handed some of the students their huge vitamin dose — staring at them until swallowed. Usually, they would hand out the pills at meal times, but not always.

I really don't know why I didn't see … Or, perhaps I just ignored the bad things I saw and heard at Narconon. When I look back, I feel guilt and sadness that I didn't stand up for those who couldn't or wouldn't protest how they were being treated.

Stuck in my memory to this day, is a young lady who fell when crossing the icy parking lot. Her arm fractured in three or four locations and she was hurting. A staff member took her to a hospital emergency ward where the attending physician ordered her to return the next day to set the fracture and apply a cast.

The physician prescribed Tylenol #3 to alleviate her pain and help her rest though the night. But the unforgiving staff refused to administer the pain medication. She was left alone to suffer through the night in agony.

I saw her crying in the dining room and sat down to ask what was wrong.

"They won't give me any of the pills the doctor gave me," she said, sobbing.

She was a dear friend and I felt so sorry for her — holding back my own tears was not easy. Not only could I feel her pain, but I was livid that anyone could intentionally allow this suffering.

I was told the next day by staff that the reason they did not administer the pain meds was that she would not be able to continue her program in the Objectives course if she was taking medication — "it was a policy."

"She won't get anything out of the course," another staff said. Again, I was confronted with these cult policies being paramount over the health of a student.

They just didn't seem to care how much pain this young lady was suffering from — 'LRH Tech' ruled over all.

Not until after I escaped did I understand that it was Scientology policy doctrine that no 'pre-clear' (student) could be on meds when receiving

A Military Compound of Surveillance and Suffering

auditing. I learned that the Narconon Objectives course was Scientology auditing sessions and that Narconon students were defined as 'pre-clears'.

As with most cults, Scientology's Narconon replaces common language with their own internal, group language. It's a complex vocabulary that redefines meanings, shuts down critical thinking, making it difficult to communicate with outsiders.

Scientology's goal is to take a person from 'pre-clear' to 'clear' and up their expensive bridge to total freedom. But we were blind. We didn't know that we were being indoctrinated with one book, one 'TR' — and one auditing session at a time.

The evil crept into us one baby step at a time on an invisible "gradient" into darkness. I was blinded by the confusion and distraught over what I saw happening to many "students".

Narconon calling ill and suffering people "students" instead of "patients" should have been a red flag to me and it still bothers me to this day.

According to L. Ron Hubbard, Narconon is "The Bridge to the Bridge" as seen in a Narconon News document that promotes Narconon as a recruiting tool for Scientolgy.

One morning I was sitting beside an executive in the dining room at breakfast when we heard a loud banging noise and yelling above us on the second floor. A young man was trying to smash down the medical officer's door with a large red fire extinguisher to get some painkillers. I remember seeing this poor guy the previous day, lying on a picnic table curled up in a fetal position. He was holding his hand against the side of his face. I was standing on the sundeck with a staff member and asked what was wrong with him. The response was, "Oh, he's just dramatizing a painful toothache and wants attention." It was horrible watching him in pain while the staff did nothing to help. Nothing!

Later that same day, an executive said to me, "David, don't be concerned about him, he's gay and below two on the Tone Scale, and a compulsive liar." Holding back my anger, I stood up and walked over to my room to diarize what had just happened. What the staff member said to justify not doing anything to help this student, who paid thousands to be cared for, pissed me off to no end.

"Don't these bastards have compassion or empathy in their hearts or soul? Do they even have a soul?" I wondered.

After things calmed down a bit, the young lad was loaded into a Narconon van and driven to a homeless shelter in Montreal, dropped off, and abandoned. This is a common practice at many Narconons. If a student is not cooperating or might cause trouble to staff and their program, the student is discarded like some piece of trash.

Another student had their prescribed medications taken away and attempted suicide by jumping out the second floor window, as my daughter described it to me after she left Narconon.

Yet another student was left unattended in the withdrawal unit and attempted suicide. According to the student's mom, Yvonne Keller, who was interviewed by CBC TV on April 9, 2012, her son "harmed himself by cutting his arms with a knife and he managed to get access to rubbing alcohol, which he drank. He was supposed to be under 24-hour supervision, which clearly he wasn't," said Keller. "An addict who is in a withdrawal unit needs to be extremely carefully supervised and I'm not sure they were capable."

A week after her son arrived at Narconon, staff rejected him from the program and put him on a bus back to Toronto, penniless and alone.

After Andre Ahern, the Narconon spokesperson, admitted to CBC TV that he was a Scientologist, he stated that Narconon uses the teachings of Scientology in its program. "She will get her money back for sure," he promised the CBC news reporter. In an email to me, Yvonne Keller said she was never paid back one cent.

Some students were disciplined with forced labour cleaning windows, dining room tables, floors, and even picking up pine cones off the ground. Others were forbidden to talk to any other student. They were only permitted to speak with certain staff members — a shunning similar to that of the Jehovah's Witnesses.

As I would pass by one person that was forced into silence, she looked down and away- glassy-eyes filled with tears. So, so sad to see and feel. I suppose the cult had more of a grip on me than I noticed, because I just went along with this like a trained puppy. Flash-backs to these events still happen today as I'm writing this, and on occasion, I struggle to hold back my tears. I witnessed similar abusive events all too often, and in a normal environment, I probably would have called authorities immediately.

Punishment and Slavery

One afternoon, a pregnant young lady who had broken one of Narconon's rules had to go through an Ethics Cycle. She was punished by being forced to shovel snow in the parking lot.

I knew who had dished out such degradation, and controlling my anger at this person was wincingly difficult. I viewed the staff culprit as a power-tripping obnoxious, baboon with an over inflated ego. In my opinion, he had accomplished very little in life, and was under the false impression that he was the high and mighty 'police officer' at Narconon.

Several of us were on the sundeck watching as she laboured — one shovel scoop after another. When she finally finished moving the big pile of snow, she smiled and walked upstairs to the 'Ethics Office'. Within minutes, she was back with shovel in hand, and began to shovel all the snow back to where she had already shovelled it from.

I spoke to her long after Narconon was shut down, and although she was traumatized and upset by the event at the time, she has now let it go. The ordeal doesn't bother her so much now, and she is doing very well — going to NA (Narcotics Anonymous) group therapy sessions to stay clean.

And again, just when I thought I had witnessed it all, one hot, sunny afternoon out on the dining room deck, a young man struggled to tell us his horrific tale of near death inside Narconon. We were standing around him on the deck — several of us stared in disbelief as we listened to what he was saying. It seemed incomprehensible that such a thing could happen.

His usual happy smile was replaced with a colorless look of sadness and wonder as a taxi pulled into the parking lot and the driver stepped out of the car. The young lad looked ill and confused.

"What's the taxi for," I asked, as the young man directed the driver to the front office.

The words unfolded as he described his trauma of being hospitalized after suffering through many days inside the blazing hot sauna and taking large doses of Niacin and other vitamin concoctions. He spent five hours a day under extreme heat conditions, but was *not* administered his prescribed insulin for an acute diabetic condition. The young man was rushed to the

Dante's Eighth Circle

hospital where the immediate attention of emergency physicians and staff saved his life. Without this emergency care, he could have easily died.

After three days in the hospital, the student phoned Narconon for a ride back. It was very late or early morning hours and nobody answered his call. So, he set out on foot to walk back, but felt too weak to keep going. So he walked back to the hospital and took a taxi to Narconon. But when they arrived, there was nobody there at the center with money to pay for the fare.

That's why the taxi driver was there at Narconon the next day — to collect his money that Narconon didn't pay the previous night.

After the young man finished his story and the taxi left, I asked him "what are you going to do now?" He replied, "I just want to leave here as soon as possible and go home." The colour in his face seemed drained of blood and his skin had a dull gray look.

As I was standing there listening to his story, I'm thinking, "Could this be true, nobody would ever NOT give someone their required insulin medication, would they?" It seemed beyond belief.

The hospital staff was so angry at the Narconon staff member who brought the student in that she broke down in tears when she later told me what happened.

I saw the young man again before he left, and as I was walking across the parking lot to my room, one of the security guards said: "David, somebody should contact the authorities before someone dies here." I think he was hoping I would do it because he sure didn't want to. As with most staff, fear of losing their job was real and silence was instilled to "keep your mouth shut or else." What could I do? I just responded that I couldn't call authorities. I told him shit would hit the fan for my Ethics Officer daughter, and that if he was so concerned, call authorities himself, "You do it," I told him. "It's your bloody job to call police or other authorities if someone is in danger or being abused." He refused and no call was made.

Many more would suffer.

The next day, an executive, Sue Chubbs, heard a few staff talking about what had happened to the young man. She walked up and said loudly, "If I hear anyone talking about this again I will pound them," and shook her fist.

A Military Compound of Surveillance and Suffering

Chubbs was well known for her robust manner, and as another staff stated in writing, "Sue was an extremist in her way of thinking. She could refuse to let someone go to the hospital because she was going to do 'Assists' on them in the withdrawal unit." She was a nasty, nasty sort to me and to others.

As usual, a very serious, life threatening incident was swept under the carpet, just like all the other crazy, abusive crap at Narconon, and no one was allowed to talk about it.

Chapter 8

Get Back in the Box

Are you kidding me — the doctor knew my condition a couple weeks after arriving here, and your telling me now?

Many of the staff and students said things like, "Oh Dave, you're going to love getting all the toxins out of your body in sauna — it's great." But when they said these things, it was with a smirk, not sincere or as if they really enjoyed it.

I was thrilled to have finished the Narconon Book 1, *Training Routines*, which one must complete before entering the sauna. But first I had to see Dina in her Qualifications office and attest to completing it. First, she had to check my 'indicators' for being cheerful and happy. If I had 'bad indicators' (sad), an interview with the Ethic's Officer or someone from Qual would take place until I had 'good' or 'very good indicators'. Scientology, LRH Tech was enforced 100% of the time.

Doing the training routines was a horrible grueling experience because of my four back surgeries that caused me pain sitting rigid-still for so long. But I was in good spirits and smiling in Dina's Qual office because it was over. She handed me a "Narconon Success" form and told me to write a story about how I felt. After Dina read it, she initialed it and attested that I had completed Book 1. Now I could start the sauna.

Every success story must point to Narconon (Hubbard), as the reason you felt good and happy. And unless you wrote a glowing script of applause to the cult, your file was shelved and advancement in the program halted until interviews and interrogations convinced you to abide by their wishes.

Even if a patient wanted to protest the program, what were they to do? Most patients have no money, no return ticket home, and cannot speak French. If the staff gets wind that someone is not happy, upset and wants to leave, their sponsor or parents are contacted immediately and manipulated into believing what is said to them from staff.

The sponsor or parent is told that so and so is having a little bit of a rough time, but this is normal and expected and that the Narconon staff can handle the situation in a few days.

"All will be well, don't worry."

"Your son or daughter will be free from drugs for life and lead a productive, happy life when they're finished the program. So, when your son or daughter calls you and tells you they want to leave for whatever reason, don't give in to their pleas and help them leave Narconon. You will only be helping them back into a life of addiction," they're told.

The staff that make these calls are very good at what they do — just like a used car salesman. It's all a con to keep the money rolling in and keeping the money 'locked-down' without having to handle demands for a refund.

The next day before entering sauna, I was called into an upstairs office and told to sit down for a talk with the so-called medical person. She said my blood tests returned positive for liver problems and that I would not be permitted to enter the sauna. "It could harm you," she said. I would have to wait a few weeks to see if my condition improved.

"Are you kidding me — the doctor knew my condition a couple weeks after arriving here, and you're telling me now? At my office visit with the Narconon doctor, he mentioned nothing about not being able to do the Narconon program — even though I gave him details about my health," I explained in anger!

I finally said: "Ok, no problem, I'll just go book a flight home today and hopefully be on my way tomorrow and go back to work — I feel quite well now."

"No, no, don't do that, just wait here, David, I'll look into this for you," she said.

A few minutes later, an executive, the infamous Sue Chubbs came into the room and told me to wait until she spoke to the doctor in Montreal. I slumped back down in the chair and waited.

Chubbs returned with a big smile on her face and said, "I just spoke to Dr. Labonte and you can start the sauna program tomorrow — I'm just waiting for him to fax a letter to me in a few minutes." But what this doctor did, violated his ethical obligations, and following a formal complaint I filed with the College of Physicians, Dr. Pierrre Labonte was banned from ever associating with Narconon again. In effect, this put all Quebec physicians on notice that servicing Narconon would land them in a heap of investigations and trouble. This was one of the first steps to have Narconon in Quebec shut down in disgrace.

After walking back to my dorm room to lie down and think, it dawned on me *why* there was a change of mind. At first it made no sense — I knew my liver would never heal without a long treatment regime under a specialist.

However, since I was paying for my Narconon program in bi-weekly instalments, if I left Narconon they would not receive further funds from me. Perhaps my wife was right on the button about Narconon being a "money grab."

"Oh well, it's only a few weeks in the hot sauna and I'll be out and onto the next books — how bad can it be," I thought.

The next day I showed up for sauna with gym shorts and towel in hand — ready to begin. There was no nurse or doctor, just a staff member to give us our pills and keep us in the hot boxes. They also checked to see if our skin had reacted to the high doses of Niacin which left bright red blotches here and there, and a burning, itchy skin.

I was handed a 50–100 mg dose of Niacin and several other pills that I swallowed including a bunch of salt tablets. After a few hours of intense heat, a group of us exited the box to eat some pieces of fruit and vegetables. We gobbled down the goodies, the staff examined us for redness, and back in the hot box we went.

And it was BLOODY HOT, with sweat dripping in streams off our head and face onto the floor. We each had a one gallon jug of cold water that we gulped from often.

There were about seventeen or so of us in three sauna rooms beside each other — females and males separated. One of the told me: "Before, when there was a mix of both sexes in each sauna, we had big troubles with sexual activity." DUH!

Dante's Eighth Circle

But still, with seventeen students and only one tiny bathroom, it was a disgusting, smelly ordeal. The high doses of vitamins caused severe diarrhea in most of the students — with symptoms of 'pissing out our burning asses' for weeks — very disgusting and painful. Some students vomited on the floor! It was not like students told me it would be — it was HELL.

Whenever we complained of pain, we were told, "Get back in the box... what turned it on will turn it off." Scientology doctrine believes that if the sauna turned on the pain or ailment, going back in the box will turn OFF the pain or cure the illness.

"What a bunch of quack bullshit," I thought, and couldn't believe their reasoning for why people became ill while enduring long, hot periods in the sauna — especially with their bellies aching with handfuls of toxic pills.

On about the 3rd day in sauna, my body had not reacted to the Niacin. No red blotches or itching. The staff member handed me a small cup of powder and told me that she had crushed the pills so that they would give me a reaction. A few minutes after swallowing the paste, my skin burned bright red and I had a terrible itching all over my body.

"Oh good, the Niacin is working," she laughed.

An hour or so later the itching had subsided and I vowed never to take any 'crushed' pills again!

After three weeks of taking huge cups of vitamins and oils, my lower abdomen began to ache terribly and I refused to take the pills all at once. I started taking them in two doses. I took one dose in the morning and one after I ate lunch. I was still in pain but able to finish the sauna program in 25-26 days when I reached 2,600 mg of Niacin.

A couple days before reaching the 2,600 mgs, I asked other students, "How the hell do I get out of here and finish this bullshit?" It was common practice for students to tell others what to say and write about different parts of the program.

"David, just write a short note called your 'end phenomena' and say that you felt terrible and confused before coming into sauna, but now you feel great physically and have a clear thinking mind," said one student who was doing the sauna for the second time.

For me, it was easy to scribble down a short note and get out of hell, but for my Twin, he was not so lucky.

Nearing the end of his sauna, he became very ill with severe pain in his abdomen. Staff tried to keep him in the sauna but he was in too much pain. He was told to go to his room and lay in bed until he felt better. He was left alone for several hours all afternoon until the pain was unbearable.

Finally, after a 'student control' staff saw he was still suffering in agony, they drove him to hospital emergency where he was admitted and treated.

I was so angry that Narconon staff allowed him to suffer all afternoon — all alone in his room with no medical care. He was not only my Twin, but also my close friend and I cared about him a lot.

Another student in the sauna suffered in pain from a swollen ankle that was later diagnosed as gout and treated by a doctor, but not before he suffered for days and endured untold agony.

Not only did many suffer from physical pains while in the sauna — the psychological trauma affected many. One young lad punched his fist through the sauna door window and another put his knuckles through the cooler window in the dining room.

Staff didn't seem to care — they just shrugged the events off as acceptable reactions to detoxing the mind and body.

One middle aged man demanded his right to see a psychiatrist but staff refused. He was eventually kicked out for not obeying rules. It was a court-ordered treatment that he be sent to Narconon. I remember well when the police car pulled into the parking lot and took him back to jail.

After I completed the sauna, I did feel better mentally, but I attribute my well-being to my time away from consuming prescription drugs. Of course, Narconon insisted it was the sauna and their incredible program that made me feel better and I had to write a success story attesting to such or go back into the box.

With no choice, I scribbled out a glowing story and once again, Dina in 'Qual' signed off for me to begin Narconon Book 3.

To this very day, I still have horrific nightmares about being in the sauna and seeing the abuse and suffering.

Chapter 9
Held Against My Will

I lost it! If Andre ever tries something like that again, he better have a fucking gun in his hand, I yelled down the hall!

I didn't know what to expect when opening Narconon Book 3, *The Learning Improvement Course*, but after a few pages, I laughed. "Are you serious?" I smiled at the course supervisor.

Apparently, Hubbard was going to teach me how to study using his 'discovered' three barriers to study technology — "Lack of Mass, Too Steep a Gradient, and Misunderstood Words." His theory was that all kinds of ill nauseating feelings happen when you don't understand and use his 'study tech'.

We didn't dare let the supervisor see us yawn or we'd be forced to 'word clear' a bunch of text. Yawning was a sign that we MUST have a word that's not understood. If caught, out came the dictionary, clearing words until the supervisor was satisfied they were understood. Simple words like 'the', 'it', and 'that' — it was the craziest crap ever!

What pissed me off more than anything was the fact that I was very able to study and easily pass a three hour real estate and sub-mortgage broker exam by the University of British Columbia. I wasn't a genius by any means, but I knew how to study well and wrote and self-published a business marketing book in the early '90s. To me, Book 3 was just a waste of time and nonsense in the first degree.

In frustration, I said to the supervisor: "This Hubbard dude sure doesn't care about our depleting forests eh?" Some pages only have a few lines of

Dante's Eighth Circle

text or a small image[1] as seen in Book 3, page 29.

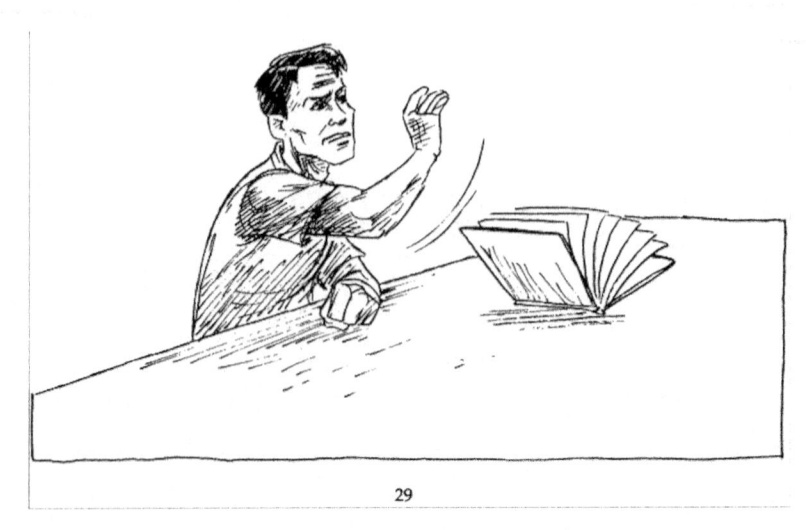

The course supervisor glared back at me without comment. I learned later that he (Phil) was a full-fledged Scientologist, and that one should not criticize L. Ron Hubbard — a god-like figure in Scientology circles.

Accused of Cheating

It only took about three days or so to finish Book 3 — then up we went to a tiny room where my Twin and I had to write a short test. There was one other student in the room writing an IQ or Personality test at the time, and we sat over at another small table in the corner.

It was a very simple and easy test and my Twin and I were laughing at some of the questions. After a few minutes the door opened and a staff member, Andre Ahern, looked in. We finished our test sheets and handed them in to Dina.

Then the 'shit hit the fan' when we were called back into Dina's office!

---

[1] Images inserted here under: 'Fair use United States law' — "Notwithstanding the provisions of sections 17 U.S.C. § 106 and 17 U.S.C. §106 A, the fair use of a copyrighted work, including such use by reproduction in copies or phonorecords or by any other means specified by that section, for purposes such as criticism, comment, news reporting, teaching (including multiple copies for classroom use), scholarship, or research, is not an infringement of copyright."

"David, Andre said he caught you guys cheating on your tests," she said.

"What the heck are you talking about? We didn't cheat — just look at our answers and compare them — you'll see we have different answers," I shot back.

"Dan (not real name of my Twin), answered his according to Book 3, and I answered mine according to what I learned in school," I said in anger.

"Ok, I'll take a look and get back to you," she said.

I was livid and couldn't believe they thought someone would need to cheat to pass that simple test of nonsense and rubbish! A while later we were called back into Dina's office.

"Yes, you're right, the answers are different, and I agree that you didn't cheat, David," she said calmly.

I was not so calm and replied, "I told you and now I want an apology from Andre for accusing us of cheating without even asking us anything about it!"

"Until he apologizes, I'm not going to do anymore Narconon books," I blurted out.

"Ok, I'll let Andre know what you want," she replied.

Even after some time passed I was still fuming mad and stood firm on not going back into the course room. The senior Ethics Officer called Dan and I up to his office and Andre was standing inside the door. He was a tall lanky kind of guy and I had experienced his heavy French accent when he went over the sauna book with me.

"Have a seat," said the Ethics Officer, John. Dan and I sat beside each other facing John across the desk as Andre stood by the door.

"Ok, what's the problem," asked John?

I replied, "I'm not going back on course until Andre apologizes for accusing us of cheating. Dina agrees we did not cheat." Then Andre said he would not apologize and went on a rant about hearing and seeing us talking.

I said, "Andre, we were not talking about the test or answers, we were chuckling and commenting about how silly the test was!" He still refused and kept *nattering* on.

I finally said, "Andre, you sound like a bloody politician the way you talk!"

Dan spoke up and said, "C'mon Andre, just apologize to Dave and we can move on."

Andre replied, "I am not going to apologize and Book 6 will handle this for David."

Of course, I had no idea what Book 6 was or what the hell Andre was talking about. In disgust, I said, "Ok, I have had enough of this crap," and stood up to walk out of the office.

Andre stood directly in front of the door with his arms up and replied, "No, you're not leaving — we're not finished here yet, so sit back down!" He stood directly in front of the door with his hands on the sides. I knew I could not leave without pushing him aside — or more like throw him out the window into a snow-bank is what I felt like doing.

He was a stubborn bastard and we would clash swords again. After a few more words from John, Andre stood aside and let us out the door.

I was fuming angry! My daughter, across the hall in her junior Ethics office could hear me cussing as we walked down the hall.

"Dad, stop making so much noise," she called out down the hall.

I lost it! "If Andre ever tries something like that again, he better have a fucking gun in his hand," I yelled down the hall!

I felt like I had just been held prisoner against my will. I knew what he had done was bullshit, illegal, and Ahern was an evil sort to be dealt with at a later time ... after I escaped the cult.

When I was free and had filed complaints with government agencies, Narconon's lawyer, Yves Rocheleau, admitted and confirmed that I was detained against my will. However, Mr. Yves Rocheleau stated that Narconon staff were justified in doing so. The lawyer said it was for my own good and stated so in a letter to me.

I was amazed to see Narconon Law Firm admit guilt. Their lawyer went on to state that Narconon was:

> Motivated, as you very well know, by your condition at the beginning of your program, which our client believes it need not describe in details at this time.
>
> Our client was responsible for your safety, particularly during what appears to have been a difficult time in your life, and it acted appro-

priately and without fault in the circumstances and at all time during your stay at its facilities.

When I read the long letter I thought, "At least they told the truth about this — too bad they lied about so many other events and abuses." I vehemently opposed the lawyer's position and responded the next day.

"There is absolutely no justification whatsoever, of illegally detaining a person against their will in any treatment facility. It is to be noted that, there is no necessity in a false imprisonment case to prove that a person used physical violence or laid hands on another person. It is sufficient to show that at any time or place the person in any manner deprived another person of his/her liberty without sufficient legal authority." The Quebec Human Rights Commission found Narconon responsible for, and guilty of, detaining me against my will. And I was not the only one to be held captive.

Another patient at Narconon Trois-Rivières was reported being held against their will, and I filed a report to the Quebec Health agency person, Denis Grenier, stating in my letter:

> On October 11, 2011, I received an email from a person in Alberta, Canada. This person is in contact with a patient who is currently at Narconon Trois-Rivières.
>
> It is alleged that this patient is being detained against her will by means of coercion, manipulation, misrepresentation, and with-holding personal property such as identification etc. Also, some forms of outside communication are now being restricted.

In my mind, I thought, "Who the hell do these Scientologists think they are? Breaking laws and violating human rights and freedoms was something they appeared to do at will, without concern for consequences." Then I read why they thought laws were of no concern to them — they were above the law or well on their way, as Hubbard stated.

> *Somebody some day will say 'this is illegal.' By then be sure the Orgs[2] say what is legal or not.* —L. Ron Hubbard[3]

---

[2] Scientology organizations
[3] Hubbard Communications Office Policy Letter, 4 January 1966, *LRH Relationship to Orgs*.

After a day or so, I cooled off and saw Andre Ahern walking towards the milk machine area. I knew that stubborn prick was not going to apologize for the life of him. I walked over to him and said, "Look Andre, I'm sorry for yelling at you down the hall, can we just let this go and get on with it?" I held out my hand and we 'kissed and made up', so to speak, and Dan and I went back on course. I just wanted OUT of Narconon as soon as possible.

To this very day, I view Andre as one of the most stubborn 'Cult-Think' and indoctrinated people I have ever met — always right and the opposite of humble.

I may have let it go at the time, "But truth and justice always wins in the end," I knew and vowed.

And of course, before moving onto Narconon Book 4a, I had to write a 'success story' for Dina in Qual. It was only a few lines to appease her and get signed off, but when I put an 'unhappy-face' curve with two dots, Dina refused to sign the form until I changed it to a 'happy-face'.

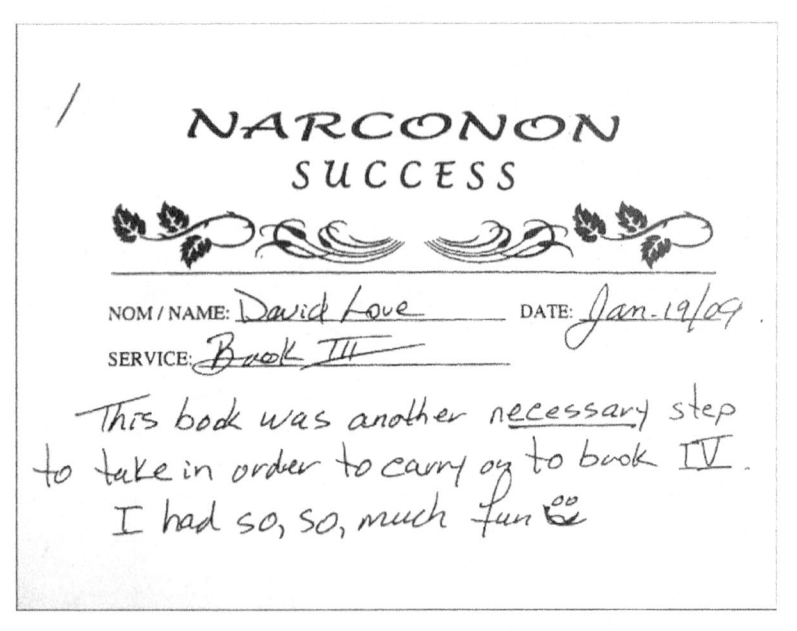

> **NARCONON SUCCESS**
>
> NOM / NAME: David Love   DATE: Jan. 19/09
> SERVICE: Book III
>
> This book was another necessary step to take in order to carry on to book IV. I had so, so, much fun 😊

Dina knew I was still not a 'happy-camper', but she let it go as 'acceptable good indicators'. And moving someone onto another phase helped raise Dina's and Narconon's all-important stats — a priority above anything else.

Chapter 10

Down the Rabbit Hole of Chaos

> *I finally figured out that not every crisis can be managed. As much as we want to keep ourselves safe, we can't protect ourselves from everything. If we want to embrace life, we also have to embrace chaos.*
> —Susan Elizabeth Phillips

The only way I can describe Narconon Book 4a is like *Alice in Wonderland's* "going down the rabbit hole" — a hellish gathering of people in chaos and confusion. I was out of sauna after doing my TRs in Book 1 with one hour sitting frozen still without moving, but now, in Book 4a the time would be doubled to two hours sitting with eyes open, and the same amount of time shut. A total of four hours sitting on a hard, rigid chair!

Again I witnessed people screaming as loud as they could at ashtrays, others frozen still in robotic stares at each other, and the most degrading, abusive insults I've ever heard. In Book 1, we bull-baited each other, but could not use any phrases concerning sex or drugs. Book 4a was a *no holds barred* game of intrusive abuse — attacking your Twin as hard as possible. The person had to remain absolutely still and not flinch or react. We could even touch their collar, and one student grabbed a student's pants zipper, pretending they would pull it open.

There were degrading insults such as: "You're nothing but a crack-whore and the court will never give you your kids back" — "You're mother doesn't know who your dad is" — "You smell like a junky, drug addict, slut and your face is ugly" — OR — "Do you put a mask on when you take a girl out" — "Your kids are not yours, I know the guy who's screwing your wife while you're in here!"

Dante's Eighth Circle

I could not believe what I was hearing. "This wasn't going to help a person stay clean and sober," I thought. Narconon staff stood off to the side laughing, as well as student onlookers — some smiling, others with strange looks on their confused faces. Even the name of Book 4a, *Communication and Perception Course*, didn't make sense. This was not 'communication' in a civil society, nor was it any recognizable 'perception' that I was used to.

The only 'perception' was using my ability to see, hear and my gut feeling of, "What the hell is going on here?" I later learned that Book 4a was Scientology Training routines and Auditing Sessions directly from their religious doctrines — gradual steps of brain washing and mind control. We were being controlled and learning to control others on command.

My Twin and I made it through Book 4a unscathed for the most part, and did laugh more than most. But I didn't know the impact these seemingly mundane drills would have on my psych and ability to sleep. I awoke many nights, soaking wet from horrible, frightening nightmares. Some demonic-like dreams I had never experienced before these cult indoctrination sessions. Yes, I had bad dreams when I first entered the dorm, but these were evil dreams of an evil, spiritual nature.

Hubbard's definition in Book 4a of 'Objectives' was: "Something real and observable ... existing outside the mind as an actual object and not merely in the mind as an idea -real." Just reading Hubbard's nonsense had me stunned. I had never read such hard to understand rubbish. Crazy!

He also said 'Objectives' is "... about outward things, not about the thoughts and feelings of the speaker." His theory is "drugs tend to push a person into experiences of the past and stick him in these experiences. Often, he is not aware that this is occurring." I viewed Hubbard's dogma as quackery. My addiction began when I was young, trying to calm the physical and mental pain from broken bones, several surgeries, and forty-three days in the hospital at age twelve — near death.

"How can I deal with or address *why* I was a drug addict if I wasn't allowed to talk about it?" I tried talking to staff and executives. "Addiction treatment and therapy isn't mind reading, it's talking," I expressed, but my voice fell on deaf ears.

Many other patients were suffering from similar agonizing pains from past years in addiction, but Narconon never once helped any of us deal with our past demons. The staff insisted we stay in 'present time' — always, no exceptions ... ever!

Narconon was beyond quackery, it was like being in a live dream that played out day after day with no end in sight.

Over at two chairs, Twins were reading from an *Alice in Wonderland* book: "It's a Cheshire cat" and "turn a somersault in the sea" while the other Twin acknowledged what was said.

"Do birds fly, and do fish swim," could be heard every day in the course room. Everything we did in Book 1, we did in Book 4a, only intensified to the max with more drills added.

I remember one shouting at an ashtray session that continued into the absurd. She was a lady who did not survive, and died soon after being kicked out of Narconon. She was a beautiful lady — loved to laugh and help others and was a dear friend.

I was her 'coach' one afternoon and the supervisor instructed me to drill her on an additional 'ashtray' process called "intention without reservation." I read from the book, instructing her to: "Think the thought — I am a wild flower." — "Good." — "Think the thought you are sitting in a chair. Good."

"Imagine that thought being in that ashtray. Imagine that ashtray containing that thought in its substance."

"Good, now get the ashtray thinking that it is an ashtray. Good. Now, get the ashtray intending to go on being an ashtray. Good." The "Yelling at an ashtray to stand up and sit back down on the chair" drill was alien all by itself. And for a few students, the 'Case Supervisor' would order this "imagine yourself being in that ashtray" crap.

Just think about it. This was nuttier than nutty — way off the edge. And this went on and on for hours, non-stop until the supervisor gave a pass!

Many of us were in the course room struggling with Book 4a for several days — morning, afternoon, and evenings until about 7 pm sometimes. Then back over at the dorm after course, students would say, "Oh, you're going to really love Book 4b Objectives — it's really going to help you change."

"Change," I asked? A few students said it helped them a lot, but they didn't say how? I remembered well what they said about the sauna being great, so I wasn't impressed with their natter about Book 4b.

Dante's Eighth Circle

In Book 1 TRs, the maximum eyes close and open was for one hour each without moving or flinching. Book 4a was four hours in total ... double the time! Two hours eyes open and two hours with eyes closed! But, this round would stretch my patience and physical endurance to my very painful limit.

My last back surgery involved removing three lumbar discs. It involved replacing the disc spaces with solid bone, titanium rods, and screws to hold all in place until the bone fused. Sitting for two hours without moving was impossible for me and I made it quite clear that I could not physically do it.

The supervisor and other staff knew that I had these surgeries, causing pain if I remained in the same position for too long. It seemed I had to battle each day with different supervisors to make them understand.

One morning, I was frustrated, in pain after sitting frozen for one hour, and still had one hour to go. The pain was too much ... shooting down my legs. In furious anger, I stood up, kicked the chair a few feet over to the side and said, "I don't give a rat's ass if you flunk me — I cannot and will not do this, so shove it where the sun don't shine — I'm done!" As I was walking out of the course room, the supervisor called out to me, "I'm sorry, David, I forgot about your back surgery." Forgetting about someone's disability and pain seemed so unprofessional and unconcerned. "Incredible," I mumbled!

An hour later after a rest on my bed, I went back to the course room with a solution in mind. I was determined they would accept my proposal or I was going home. I would not accept their compromises.

I had made up my mind, "It's either my way, or the highway, baby! Enough is enough and I had had enough of their bullshit to last a lifetime and more." So, I suggested, "Look, there is only one way I will be able to complete these two hours of TRs non-stop. Let's break the 120 minutes down into three segments of forty minutes each. I only need to stand up after each forty minutes and stretch a bit, then do the next forty minutes at a time until we're done." The supervisor replied that she would have to pass it by Marc Bernard, the Case Supervisor at the time, but she viewed my suggestion as doable if Marc agreed.

If I was to try to explain Book 4a in a few words to someone on the outside, it would be nearly impossible. I said to one student: "If a doctor, nurse or a qualified addiction therapist ever walked into this course room, they would think we were all crazy and have the place shut down immediately." L. Ron Hubbard's written instruction to a course room Supervisor: "If there are too many questions from a student, send him to Review," meaning to the Qualifications Office or Ethics Officer if appropriate. Students knew that this was the case as described on page 407 of Book 1. So, most students avoided asking questions about things they didn't understand.

One afternoon I was in the Qual office with tears running down my face and Sue Chubbs came into the office. "David where is *that* all coming from," she asked rudely.

I replied, "What do you mean, where is *that* coming from," wondering why she was so cold.

"David, you need to get back in 'present time' and out of your past," she blurted out.

She was one of the coldest women I had ever met. I discovered much later that she was a Scientologist, and followed Hubbard's so-called technology to the tee. But also, Chubbs was viewed by many as a ruthless bitch by both staff and students, and students blurted out descriptions of her that are too obscene to publish here.

As there were no councillors at Narconon that I could talk to about my anguish, I just had to hold my pain inside and press on. 'Present Time' was not something I stayed in often — past turmoil kept dragging me back.

Chapter *11*

Hacking into Souls

> *It makes Dr. Fu Manchu look like a kindergarten student. It is the ultimate vampirism, the ultimate mind fuck. Instead of going for blood, you're going for their soul.*
>
> *But, of course, it takes a couple of hundred hours of auditing and mega thousands of dollars for the privilege of having your head turned into a glass Humpty Dumpty — shattered into a million pieces.* —L. Ron Hubbard Jr.

The big day arrives, and we enter the world of Scientology auditing sessions ... opening course Book 4b — 537 pages designed to hack into and crack your soul.

To save money, Narconon teaches each student how to run each other through these mind altering sessions. They taught us how to fill out the 'Session Report Forms' and 'Worksheets' and they gave us giant teddy bears to practice with.

We sat the fuzzy teddy on our laps and used our ventriloquist voices to have the bear speak while moving its paws in gestures. My Twin and I laughed continuously it was so ridiculously funny.

Dante's Eighth Circle

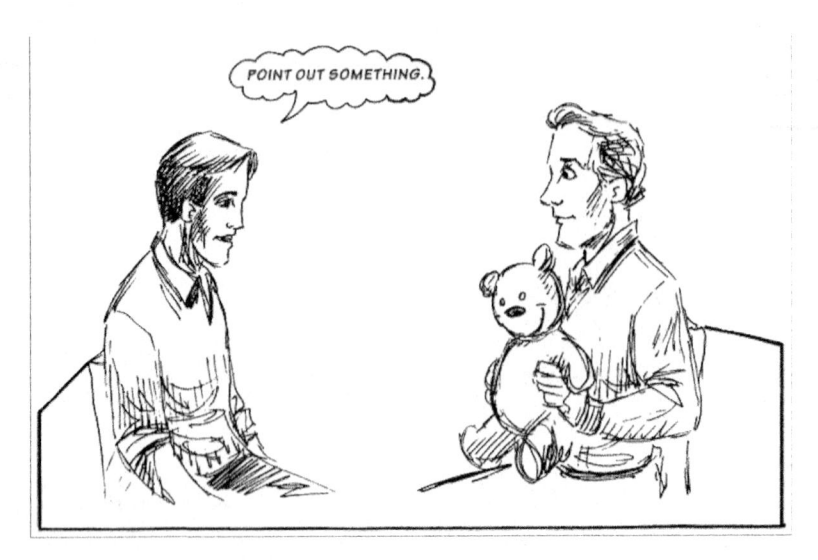

POINT OUT SOMETHING.

Now, when I think about this practice of using rehab patients to treat each other, and not hiring qualified staff to do so, I shudder. I can't imagine any other reputable treatment center even considering such a thing. But then again, this was not science based treatment — we were deep inside the dark throat of an evil cult.

Once we passed the teddy bear test, the course supervisor allowed us to begin sessions on each other.

Book 4b lasted about six long weeks, and I viewed the material and actions as being medieval torture — forced to do things contrary to my beliefs. Unknown to me at the time, the calculating staff were engaged in practices to alter my reasoning and thoughts, and distort my own sense of values. It was Hubbard 'Tech' all the way or the student was kicked out and sent down the highway.

Each morning I would wake up, and remember vivid, horrible dreams. I'd drag my frustrations out of bed, knowing that I faced another day of being presented with new information that I would have to learn through repetitive routines and drills. On several occasions I would leave the course room in anger and go back to my room — "A mental ward would be saner than this place," I thought!

Whenever I complained or balked at the course materials, I was sent for "word-clearing" drills, and on one occasion, had to endure a "False Data Stripping" process.

False data stripping consisted of handling my so-called antagonism. It was a process that was Hubbard's way of telling Scientologists to disregard any sources of information which Hubbard himself disagreed with. If what I thought or spoke out was contrary to Hubbard's text, it was false data information, and this cult wanted my mind stripped of what I thought and believed was true.

I constantly called into question what the material I was studying had to do with drug addiction treatment or therapy. None of the course supervisors would give me a direct answer, always pointing me back to the course book.

They told me false data stripping was the answer to me understanding and learning the material. Their attempt to trick me into believing something other than what I knew was true made me angry. I refused to continue the process. The Qualifications and Ethics Officer's interrogations didn't help, and only frustrated me to my limit.

On one afternoon, I was walking up the stairs out of the course room and saw several people in the stairwell. They were facing the wall with a sheet of paper in their hand, memorizing the 12 Social and 12 Anti-Social attributes. One was repeating stuff to a supervisor verbatim and I shook my head, wondering… "Why was this silliness so important?" I would learn soon enough that Narconon took these attributes very seriously and we would soon clash opinions once again — battling my beliefs against theirs.

Hubbard dogma[1] states:

> Don't be surprised if physical reactions such as body twitches, tiredness and pains turn on while doing these Objectives. The person receiving them might also get sad or angry. These are signs that changes are occurring with a person in the session. Just continue doing the Objective.

Every time I said to the supervisor, "I'm done this session and ready to move onto the next," he would respond with, "No just keep going." One of our first sessions continued on for an entire week non-stop. I felt like I was losing my mind. It was so draining… so exhausting that we became sleepy — our eyes heavy and ready to close and drift off. The repetitions of "do this and do that… look there and walk" were hypnotic.

On page 165 it began —

---
[1] Narconon program books

Dante's Eighth Circle

1. "YOU LOOK AT THAT WALL" — "THANK YOU"

2. "YOU WALK OVER TO THAT WALL" — "THANK YOU"

3. "YOU TOUCH THAT WALL" — "THANK YOU"

4. "TURN AROUND" — "THANK YOU"

An entire week of these exhausting, crazy sessions did something to me, twisting inside my mind. And hours on end of ...

1. "LOOK AROUND HERE AND FIND SOMETHING THAT IS REALLY REAL TO YOU"

2. "LOOK AROUND HERE AND FIND SOMETHING YOU WOULDN'T MIND COMMUNICATING WITH"

3. "LOOK AROUND HERE AND FIND SOMETHING YOU WOULDN'T MIND BEING AROUND."

At first glance, from an outsider's perspective, one might think that this is a simple enough exercise. And indeed it is, but the repetition of hearing the stern commands, and having to obey them without question or reaction is what twisted my mind. The repetition and duplication over and over again was Scientology's cult processes of mind control in gradients of tiny steps.

There was a Scientology handbook in the student file cabinet that one supervisor would take out and read certain passages to see if the student was "CRACKED." L. Ron Hubbard, Jr. once said to an interviewer about Scientology:

> Brainwashing is nothing compared to it. The proper term would be "soul cracking."

> It's like cracking open the soul, which then opens various doors to the power that exists, the satanic and demonic powers. Simply put, it's like a tunnel or an avenue or a doorway. Pulling that power into yourself through another person and using women, especially is incredibly insidious.

Hacking into Souls

It makes Dr. Fu Manchu look like a kindergarten student. It is the ultimate vampirism, the ultimate mind fuck. Instead of going for blood, you're going for their soul. And you take drugs in order to reach that state where you can, quite literally, like a psychic hammer, break their soul, and pull the power through.

He designed his Scientology Operating Thetan techniques (Scientology's secret initiations) to do the same thing. But, of course, it takes a couple of hundred hours of auditing and mega thousands of dollars for the privilege of having your head turned into a glass Humpty Dumpty — shattered into a million pieces. It may sound like incredible gibberish, but it made my father a fortune.

Any doubts I expressed about the teachings was my fault, and never a Hubbard mistake or Narconon's fault. Negativism toward the session was misdirected back to me — causing me to internalize my doubts. I imagined I was living in a frozen hell on earth — my obedience to stern commands had me mentally tied in angry knots of distress.

My past experiences and values were invalid if they conflicted with what Narconon was teaching. My views had no value and deemed insignificant when compared to the value of the group. Group belief superseded my individual conscience and integrity as I struggled on.

While revisiting the horrors at Narconon while writing this book, the traumatic pain resurfaces from horrific events. To this day I still suffer from physician diagnosed Post-Traumatic Stress Disorder (PTSD), struggling daily to unwind the knotted mess created by evil.

Five weeks, six days per week of 'Training Routines' and auditing sessions, have embedded unwanted thoughts. The commands of "give me that hand, touch that wall, touch that chair, touch your nose," and on and on — seemingly forever, changed me.

We were in a large room for Book 4b Objectives. It used to be the Catholic Church worship room for the Nuns — now turned into a cult of Scientology indoctrination den. Folding tables were set up near the outside walls, leaving room for other sessions to be done in other areas.

Some students were sobbing in tears — one was crawling around the floor on his hands and knees. A few were nodding off and even I went into a hypnotic type state — asleep, but my head was up while my Twin was moving my hand around as we sat at a table.

You really had to be there to really know and understand what is so difficult to put into words. It would be similar to when my very young son burned his hand on our wooden stove. We told him several times, "Do not touch the stove, its HOT" ... but he had to see and feel for himself — screaming and crying in pain for hours. Once he experienced the real pain, he knew exactly what we meant.

The man who was crawling around on the floor didn't attend his graduation ceremony at Friday's weekly event. He was too messed up. But he did write the craziest speech for director Marc Bernard to read to the crowd.

Marc stood on the stage behind the 'pulpit' and said he was handed a script from Shane (not real name), and agreed to read it for him.

The speech was ONE word only, in groups of one, two, and three etc. that went something like this:

"Meow, meow-meow-meow, meow-meow, meow, meow-meow, meow-meow-meow, meow," that went on for a few minutes. Marc commented that he was only reading it because he gave his word he would.

I was stunned, as were all the others listening to Marc read this most ridiculous speech ever heard. It should go down in history as, "What is Scientology, and how does Scientology auditing affect those who do not know they are being brain-washed and soul-cracked." Perhaps "All the King's horses and all the King's men couldn't put Humpty Dumpty together again," may be more real than one could imagine. Many patients, after leaving Narconon, are far worse off than when they entered the cult rehab. Some require years of therapy to deprogram from the psychological mind intrusion — twisting once functional adults into mere broken souls.

Shane was a nice guy from the Far East, and we spent a lot of time discussing our religious beliefs and philosophy. He also bought a thick book about Scientology that he would bring into the dining room to read and show me.

One day a staff member picked up the book and told Shane he couldn't have it at Narconon. Later, I asked Shane "why" and he replied that he wasn't really sure. He eventually ended up going through an 'ethics cycle' for something he had done, and I could see he was changing — not his usual happy self. He seemed robbed of his inner joy he had expressed so often. It was so sad to see.

We kept in contact for a while after he graduated while I was on staff, but I haven't heard from him in quite some time now. From some of his past Facebook posts, it appears he still praised Narconon as his saviour after he left.

As I progressed through Book 4b, I grew more frustrated every day, wondering when this hell was going to end.

Many times I would argue with the supervisor or refuse to 'cooperate' as they defined my refusal. In one of the Objectives sessions I was commanded the ridiculous. "Look at that wall — Walk over to that wall — Touch that wall." So far so good — "No problem, I thought." Then the crazy command of "Keep it from going away — and did you keep it from going away," stopped me in my tracks.

"Huh, what is this about — of course I can't keep a wall from 'going away' — it's not a living object that can move or walk away," I said.

So every time my Twin repeated the commands, I would say, "NO, I didn't keep it from going away!" Dan, my Twin, walked over to the supervisor and said, "David is not going to say yes no matter how long we keep doing this." The supervisor told him to "Keep going with the commands." After another hour or so, I walked over to the supervisor and said, "I'm not going to say yes to stopping that wall from moving — it does not have a will and it's not moving on its own. It's not going away all by itself, so how am I stopping it?" Like most of the Narconon program, it didn't make sense and the staff was not allowed to explain or express their opinion of 'why' or 'how'.

After a time, I agreed to say "yes," but told the supervisor in blunt terms, that I did NOT believe I had stopped that wall from going away.

I now understand why Shane was crawling around on his hands and knees and his graduation speech was "meow" only.

In some of the Objective sessions I was commanded like a dog in training, "Walk over there — Stop — Walk over to that letter on the floor." The repetitious demands had me obeying without question — like putty in Hubbard's hands.

However, I was not finished my objections to their 'Objectives' yet, and the last session was about to cause the staff some of their own distress.

The last exercise was called, "Book and Bottle." About 8-10 feet apart was placed a blue book, "The Way to Happiness" on a table, and a green wine bottle on a window sill. I was commanded to "Look at that book — Walk over to it — Pick it up — What is its color — What is its temperature — What is its weight — Put it down in exactly the same place." Sounds simple enough to me — no problem until I asked myself, "How the hell do I know what the bottle weighs or what the temperature is?" This was not a one or two hour session, but went on for many hours into three full days!

On the third day of picking up the bottle, I yelled, "What the hell is this bullshit all about — do I look like a fricking thermometer?" I told my Twin I had enough of this crap and walked over to my room.

I told Security to get my wallet and ID immediately and I was leaving. A few minutes later, John, the scruffy senior Ethics Officer came to my room for a chat. He looked like he had been partying all night with puffy, red eyes. He was a party-boy.

He nattered on about this and that — trying the guilt trip if I left, but I told him he had no idea what he was talking about and that I was leaving for home back in B. C. no matter what he said. He even said I should stay or my daughter would be upset and stressed out if I left. I told him to leave my room and do what I asked — "Get me my wallet and ID so I can leave." Finally in frustration, he left my room and called Charles in Qualifications to meet with and talk to me. By that time, I had cooled down a bit and listened to what he said. I ended up agreeing to stay for the benefit of my Twin and daughter, not for myself.

Back in the course room for a couple more hours, and the supervisor gave me a pass and Book 4b was done. I felt so relieved I had finished six weeks of hell in Book 4b that I actually had a wide smile because it was over with. Not because I learned anything about life or about drug addiction and how to remain drug free, but because I was able to express my integrity and feelings to staff without fear. I felt violated in many aspects, but felt I could still be ME and not someone they wanted me to be.

Near the end of Book 4b, there are three or four pages devoted to Hubbard's lifelong accomplishments. Apparently he was a 'seasoned traveller', 'free-lance reporter', 'pilot', and conducted studies in drug addiction cures.

Most impressive, was Hubbard's statement that "Narconon has been setting the pace in the field of drug rehabilitation, (per independent studies), and a 70 to 80 percent success rate in helping people to come off drugs — and stay off them." — L. Ron Hubbard: Book 4b, page 553.

Even after being away from the cult of Narconon for over three years now, my mind still wanders back — viewing films in my head of the hell I and others went through. Sometimes I see the 'movie-like' scenes clearly, but other times when least expected, my mind goes dark like the power being cut to an old 8 mm projector.

And although they may have invaded my mind, twisted my thoughts that resulted in demonic nightmares, I refused to let them break, crack me, or mess with my soul. Still, the cult indoctrination had changed something in me — I could feel it like a sour taste in my mouth.

Chapter *12*

Free Time Watching the Sickness

The scene was so chaotic that the prison staff handcuffed both the student and the Narconon Ethics Officer.

Not every hour was consumed with indoctrination — we did have our free time during the week after course and all day off on Sundays for fun and games.

When living in such close quarters — lacking professional supervision, it's a diverse and sometimes chaotic stage of players. Some students and staff cross the line of sexual adventure. For some, sexual activity negatively affected them — with bad dreams and trauma while at Narconon, and for years after leaving.

Some of the female patients feared going to the Withdrawal Unit for assists because they knew of the inappropriate touching and other abuses by a staff member. In other drug rehabs, a female patient being left alone in a room with a man for a massage would never be permitted at any time. But Narconon wasn't one of your 'normal' drug rehabs — it's a cult. We referred to it as a "generating revenue machine" for Scientology.

"We save lives," is their motto. "We are a social betterment group to clear the planet of crime and drugs," and "We're the best" according to Scientologist John Travolta.

After I escaped Narconon, I received many emails from students, saying that a male withdrawal specialist had crossed the line with their touch assists. They explained that, whenever they knew this pervert was on duty in withdrawal, they would avoid going. I remember him, and the morning he was fired for inappropriate behaviour.

There were few dull moments at this Narconon center — there was always something going on that had me writing about it in my room.

No fences surrounding the large compound and the forest provided privacy for many lovers. Some couples would sneak under the pool table in the recreation room and other places for romance. There simply was not enough qualified staff to monitor all the action ... and Narconon executives appeared not to care. They only wanted to know who, where, and when for some odd reason.

A rogue Narconon ... Bring the money and we can cure you — Narconon didn't "treat" only addicts and alcoholics, but also patients suffering from bulimia or anorexia. As long as a check was delivered upon being admitted, everyone was welcome it seemed. We even had one who was a "huffer" — an addict who inhales chemical or gasoline vapours to get high. And there was a massive supply of product at Narconon.

While sitting one evening with a female student in the dining room at dinner time, I could not believe how much she was eating. It was incredible! She'd leave for a brief period, then come back and eat another huge plate of food.

She was funny and we would laugh so hard sometimes that tears would run down our faces. But, I was concerned and asked around about her possibly being bulimic. Sadly, the answer was yes. There was no counselling for her at Narconon to deal with her serious illness — only the same cookie-cutter, Scientology crap.

The most disturbing case was a skeleton of a lady who was a severe anorexic. She was so thin and gaunt that one of the female case supervisors was in shock and had emotional difficulty visiting her in the withdrawal unit. The case supervisor said, "David, I have never seen such a mess of a person in all my life, and I feel sick when talking to her." While standing on the sundeck one afternoon, I looked over and saw a couple of ladies lying on towels, sunbathing. The grass was a few inches high, and as I looked closer, there was a third person, barely visible. It was the young lady who was suffering from starvation. Narconon had been advised by its Medical Manager, Dr. Labonte, to keep a close eye on this patient because she could die if she didn't begin eating soon.

A few days later, I saw her in the Course Room doing TRs. "Oh my God," I thought, "What is this person doing at Narconon?" She needed immediate medical care. But no, they had her sit frozen still doing Scientology TRs. I could see her bones poking out beneath her pallid skin — it was horrible to see. She moved and walked in slow motion and had difficulty climbing the stairs to exit the course room.

One middle-aged man, who pleaded with staff to make him an appointment to see a psychiatrist, was refused. At that time, I was unaware of the cult's views on mental illness, so the refusal was quite astonishing to me. The patient was in obvious anguish and needed professional medical care. Finally, the staff called the local police, and he was taken away in handcuffs to jail … never to return.

Another young man in his twenties appeared one afternoon — walking around the compound grounds picking up dirt and eating it! I could see him talking to the air in an obvious psychotic state. He was a mess! Security and Student Control followed him around the grounds for quite a while watching him.

Finally, the senior Ethics Officer, John, grabbed the student and took him over to the large prison across the street from Narconon. I don't know what John was thinking? This was not a police station or hospital where the student 'should' have been taken to, it was a provincial prison.

This scene caused so much chaos when the two arrived, that the guards handcuffed both the student and the Ethics Officer.

One of the Narconon executives had to walk over to the prison to explain that one of the two detainees was a Narconon staff member and have him released.

Because the patient was in a psychotic state, he was released and taken to a local motel room, guarded by a Narconon staff. One of the guards at the motel was a student who had just graduated from the program and was in training to be a new Ethics Officer.

The latter was my room-mate in the staff quarters below the withdrawal unit. When he was off his guard shift at the motel, he would tell me stories about this poor lad's condition. The patient was delusional, hallucinating, and muttering nonsense about space aliens and invisible powers he possessed.

To me, it sounded like the student was possessed — like in the movie, 'The Exorcist'.

I wondered what qualified Narconon to keep this guy captive for the duration of his withdrawal from 'Special K' — especially in a motel room. I later learned that 'Special K' (ketamine) distorts perceptions of sights and sounds and makes the user feel disconnected and not in control. In chronic cases of ketamine dependency, the effects of the drug take from several months to a few years to wear off completely, and professional medical care is required.

Eventually the 'Special K' guy was sent for further withdrawal and detox in the United States. He later returned to complete and graduate Narconon.

While reviewing some diarized notes in my dorm room one evening, I heard a commotion downstairs and then a loud knock on my door. "David — David — come downstairs quick! Withdrawal needs your help!" I put away my notebook and followed Security down into the withdrawal unit. The withdrawal specialist was distraught and in a panicked state.

"David, this girl is really messed up, and I don't know what to do with her. She's very sick and in a lot of pain and suffering," she said in desperation. "Can you help us please?" I replied: "I'm not staff, I'm a student myself. What do you want or expect me to do?"

"David, you know how she's feeling and she will trust you. Please talk to her." I walked out into the hall and there she was — this tiny, frail young lady, leaning against the door jamb. "Oh my God," I thought, "she could die here in withdrawal. This poor soul could very well draw her last breath any minute." Forcing a half-smile and trying not to let tears flow from my wet eyes, I walked over and said, "Hello, my name is David Love. Would you like to go out on the deck and talk?" She replied, "I know who you are. Yes, I would like to talk, but I'm so cold, and I feel like dying." 'Angel' (not her real name) was so weak that she needed something to lean on to stand up. Her arms and legs were covered with dark track marks and bruises from too many days, months, and years of pain-numbing addiction.

Angel went into her room and put on a coat while I grabbed a couple of blankets to keep her from shivering so much. We chatted about how she was feeling and about my time in withdrawal. But what concerned me most were Angel's feelings of worthlessness and her not caring if she lived or died. She had a photo album, and she showed me pictures of her modeling poses and of her sweet, dear little baby girl. Her face widened in a big smile while she stared at her beautiful baby.

She was only a couple of days into opiate withdrawal, but the agony was taking a devastating toll on her already weak body and mind. I knew it was only a matter of time for her to begin feeling human again, but, that would take a few more days yet. The only thing I could do for her was just listen with a caring and compassionate heart. I explained that she was valuable and had just as much worth as any other person — and a very special value to her daughter. She began to cry and sob, wrapping her tiny arms around me for a hug. Now she had me in tears, and our close bond began.

Over the next few days, I would go down and visit 'Angel'. The staff thanked me, but I wasn't very polite to them. I considered this incompetent health care from Narconon that didn't have a clue what the fuck they were doing. TRs, Light Objectives, and Nerve Assists were not what this desperate soul needed. She needed a professional therapist and counsellor, something I was not.

One morning I walked through the dining room, and saw one of the withdrawal specialists sitting at a table with someone from the Montreal Church of Scientology. There were no smiles, only rather stern and timid looks.

'Angel' was just out of withdrawal, and she came up to me in the dining room and said, "David, I don't want to see that guy ever again. I feel sick just seeing him."

"Why?" I asked.

"Because, when I was in withdrawal, he took pictures of me and put his hands on me. It was horrible!" I told 'Angel' to leave the dining room, and I would look into it right away.

After the two men at the table finished talking, I walked up to the Scientologist, Charles, and said, "What the fuck is going on here? The police and social services should be called right now. What that pervert did to her is a criminal offence and you know it!"

"Calm down, David," he said. "We will handle this." Charles then told me the pictures were deleted from the digital camera, and the offender was being fired. But, as far as I was concerned, firing him was not good enough.

Dante's Eighth Circle

"How many others did that pervert sexually abuse or touch inappropriately." I wondered.

The Narconon abuses were definitely not limited to unwanted touching and forcing one to perform outlandish acts in the course rooms.

Some patients who broke the rules were forced into total silence and manual slave labour on orders from the Ethics Officer. A yellow poster (goldenrod) was tacked to the dining room wall for all the patients and staff to read about their "Treason and Crimes". Even though student/patient information was supposed to be confidential, the poster detailed their information for all to see and read.

For their punishment, some were not allowed to speak one word to any of their friends and some worked for days on end in humiliation. They weren't even permitted to smile at another student, and some could be seen with tears running down their cheeks as they worked.

These shunning actions affected many students well after they graduated Narconon and arrived home.

After escaping Narconon, I received an email from a sister of a young female student. She said her sister stayed in her room for months after returning home — too afraid to come out and face the real world.

There were so many disturbing events that still have a distressing effect on me today whenever I reflect back to the pain and suffering — concerning the many 'things that should not be.'

Chapter 13

Roller-Coastering: Ups and Downs in Life Disaster

Just because I get "something" caught in my zipper, doesn't mean I'm in a PTS condition — it means I was in hurry!

Narconon Book 5, *Ups & Downs in Life Course*, was another introduction into Scientology dogma that had my program halted ... stopped dead for three days and my case file shelved.

The day started, as usual, by doing a few TRs, then into the course books. On page 8 of Book 5, it seemed interesting to me that perhaps Hubbard had something I could use. Of course I wanted to be happier, a more stable person, and at first, I was interested in what this Book was about.

According to Hubbard there are only two types of personalities — the 'social' and the 'anti-social'. Good people and bad people — no in between or gray areas are considered.

I thumbed through some pages and called the course supervisor over to my course room table. As I had done several times, I asked, "What the hell does this have to do with drug addiction and treatment?" I pointed to pages 124–126 that showed a photo of Hitler saluting on one page and a total of only four sentences on the other two pages. And I once again added, "Hubbard sure didn't give a damn about the environment by saving trees — who the hell only prints one short sentence on a whole page?"

"Just keep reading, David — are there any words you don't understand?" chirped the supervisor.

I replied, "No, I understand all the words, but not *why* I am studying this crap!" Hubbard was firm on there being ONLY two types of people. To this very day, I still don't understand his quote: "So there are cowboys in white hats and cowboys in black hats. And the cowboys in the gray hats are too sick to be in the game." I still scratch my head wondering why some 'white hats' were drug addicts and some 'black hats' were clean and sober? According to L. Ron Hubbard policy, I am now a "Suppressive Person" and wearing a 'black hat'. The difference is, I am drug free now, so he was DEAD WRONG ... AGAIN!

Hubbard describes an anti-social person as a 'Suppressive Person' (SP) — a person who seeks to suppress, or squash, any betterment activity or group. A suppressive person suppresses other people in his vicinity. This is the person whose behaviour is calculated to be disastrous.

I found Hubbard's solution to suppressive persons very crazy and disturbing. He suggests that: "If society were to recognize this personality type as a sick being, as they now isolate people with smallpox, both social and economic recoveries could occur." Perhaps L. Ron Hubbard was the author of, or similar to, the real "Flying Monkey" — someone who does the narcissist's bidding to inflict additional torment to the narcissist's victim. Narconon staff was spying on the students, spreading gossip, threatening students and accusing them of being perpetrators of chaos — when in reality, the students were the unwary pawns in their 'Game.'

Of course all these book pages tugged me along on a gradient that was interesting but what I didn't see, at the time, was that I was being bamboozled into cult dogma thinking. I had to use a 'Demo Kit' to show I understood, but I really didn't at the time. I was just doing what I thought they wanted me to show.

"Roller-Coasting" was another word thrown about by staff referring to me doing very well, learning well and then plummeting into a sudden steep decline — a clear indicator to them of me being PTS. Not understanding this at first, I was offended by the label and told them off. It didn't make any sense to me whatsoever. I often tried to encourage others and raise their self-esteem, so surely I was not a suppressive person and I knew of nobody else who was. At least this is what I thought at the time.

But it turns out the term has a unconventional meaning, as is the case with much of Hubbard's made up jargon. Hubbard insists that any person, who is in contact with a Suppressive Person, is a 'Potential Trouble Source' or 'PTS'. Because I was, as Hubbard calls it, 'Roller Coastering', it was determined by staff that I was a 'Potential Trouble Source'. According to them, this 'PTS' condition was not my fault and could be cured.

Then to add to the confusion, the battle hammer of hell fell with page 228 and the L. Ron Hubbard doctrines of what causes ALL accidents and ALL illness. I still have nightmares, flashing back to the battles we had over this. I refused to believe or accept the strict dogma of L. Ron Hubbard:

> ALL ILLNESS, IN GREATER OR LESSER DEGREE, AND, ALL FOUL-UPS STEM DIRECTLY AND ONLY FROM A PTS CONDITION.

Not only was I forced to memorize all twenty-four traits of the social and anti-social personalities, but now it was insisted that I believe this rubbish! I was like an elephant on the edge of a cliff that refused to obey a command to jump off and fly. The supervisor insisted, "David, you don't have to believe it, just memorize and repeat it back verbatim."

I vehemently objected, saying, "There is no way in creation I will accept or memorize this and that's all there is to it, so let's move onto the next assignment!" But the course supervisor could not allow anything to be skipped or they would face severe disciple or even be fired. I pulled out my sword of resistance and the cult pulled out their sword of manipulation and coercion. The battle lines were drawn!

I was being forced into accepting something other than what science had proven to me in school, and agree to something with no scientific basis. Not surprisingly, I was sent upstairs to see Charles in the Qual office. "So, what's the problem this time, David," asked Charles in a serious tone. He knew I was pissed and would stand my ground on this issue as I had done on previous occasions with other rubbish and abuses.

"Listen there is no way in hell I will agree to memorize that bullshit Hubbard trash, when I know science has proven otherwise," I said.

"C'mon Charles, disease, illness and accidents are *not* caused *only* because I'm in contact with a suppressive person. Are you telling me that if I'm riding a bicycle down a gravel mountain road and have an accident because of a flat tire, that this is because I have a friend who is antagonistic to Narconon? Think about how ridiculous this theory sounds," I said.

Charles tried to explain that an accident or illness might not seem like it's connected to being in a PTS condition, but there are lots of things we don't understand at first he explained.

"Well then, explain it to me!" I was getting angrier by the minute at this nonsense. "What about germs, viruses, asbestos, and other environmental issues that cause illness and disease — are you saying *all* of these are *only* caused by me being in a PTS condition to a Suppressive Person?!" I was so angry I walked out of the office, intentionally slamming the door before heading off to the men's dorm to diarize notes about this battle.

Day two of having my program stopped was a day of psychological warfare that I vowed not to lose. In the dining room that morning during breakfast, staff asked me if I was going back on course or still refusing to complete the PTS section. I just shook my head and said, "Nope, not doing it," and went back to my room.

A while later, I was called back up to the executive office wing for more persuasion attempts. I could not understand why this concept was so important to them. It made no sense.

On the third day of arguments and angry replies from me, I again threatened to leave and go home. He insisted again that I didn't have to believe it, just memorize and repeat back to the supervisor.

I replied, "Look Charles, I am not going to inject and imprint something into my mind that I know is rubbish with no scientific basis just because somebody tells me I must do it." We chatted some more about stress and immune systems and I agreed that undue stress can weaken the immune system and cause our bodies to be more susceptible to becoming sick when germs or viruses enter our bodies. I could see where Charles was attempting to lead me and shot back in frustration.

"Just because I get my dick caught in my zipper, doesn't mean I'm in a PTS condition. It means I was in hurry or whatever!" I slammed back at Charles.

I kept up the pressure on the predominant words <u>all</u> and <u>only</u> in the context of

> All illness, in greater or lesser degree, and, <u>all</u> foul-ups stem directly and <u>only</u> from a PTS condition.

Charles looked very frustrated with me, but his sense of humour had him grin a few times and he even gave a few quiet chuckles at what I was saying. During that time period, I had very little knowledge about Scientology structure, religious doctrines, or policies. My persistence to have Charles accept my views and suggestions, to simply skip this part of the Narconon course book fell on deaf ears.

"Why is this prick being so stubborn?" I thought. Finally, after hours of speaking our minds, I said, "Ok, let's just agree to disagree on this matter and move on or I'm out of here tomorrow."

Charles knew I was paying my program fees on a bi-weekly basis and if I left, so would my money. At this point, Charles played his *hole card*. He brought up that my daughter was on staff as a junior Ethics Officer. He said that I would be letting her down, if I walked out. Although my view of Charles immediately changed to seeing him as a manipulative, cult indoctrinated bastard, I knew exactly what he meant.

We discussed integrity and other moral issues for a few more minutes and I looked him straight in the eye and said, "I'm going to give you a take it or leave it suggestion. Either you accept my proposal or I'm booking a flight home today! I will agree to repeat back to the supervisor this and this only:

ILLNESS, IN GREATER OR LESSER DEGREE AND FOUL-UPS STEM DIRECTLY AND FROM A PTS CONDITION.

"I will delete <u>all</u> and <u>only</u> — and will not say those words. Take it or leave it," I said.

Charles shook his head, smiled and said, "Ok fine. Now get back into the course room." I was still memorizing some of what I didn't believe, but I only had a few more books to finish and I could go home soon. "And these asshole Scientology pressure cookers can go screw themselves," I thought. I had never experienced such quackery in all my life, and would soon be immersed in more extreme Scientology practices, including Ethics Cycles and battles with staff.

A few days later I woke up with a simple cold. Other staff and students had colds and I caught the same bug. But the staff determined that I was PTS and sent me to the Ethics office convinced I was connected to a Suppressive

Dante's Eighth Circle

Person on the outside. They insisted the only reason I had a cold was because I was PTS.

Sitting across from the Ethics Officer, I commented, "Are you kidding me? This is crazy. I have a cold because I caught it from somebody else here who has a cold." They remembered, and brought up the phone call I received from a family member who told me Narconon was only a money grab. This was the Suppressive Person who caused my cold. "Yup, this person is only a few thousand miles away, and these super-cold viruses can fly like a bat out of hell right into me," I mused.

I was badgered about when I last had a cold, where was I, who was I with, and on and on until I stood up said, "Well, I'm going to take a mouthful of vitamin C and get rid of this sucker. Have a nice day," and I walked out in disgust! As far as I was concerned, they could shove it where the sun don't shine if they wanted me to 'handle' or 'disconnect' from a person they thought was causing my cold.

I thank God for my strong Christian beliefs. Without my faith, I really think I would have succumbed to complete conversion over to the cult of Scientology. As it was, I was talking the talk and starting to robotically behave like I was part of their group and belonged to it some sad way.

As every day passed, I would witness abusive actions — not only against the students, but also by staff against other staff members. It would be painful to hear and see. My intuition was telling me something was very wrong here. This kept me from falling over the edge into the abyss of no return.

Chapter 14

Confessions used to Attack their Enemy

> *And ... the gall of "master" Hubbard to be writing such demands, when he himself was the opposite including being married to two wives at the same time, is beyond belief!*

Narconon Book 6, *Personal Values and Integrity Course*, is something I now see as counter to what Scientology actually practices. On the one hand, Scientologists imagine themselves to be the most ethical people on the planet, when in fact, their prime directive is the survival of their *own* group, by any means necessary.

After a few pages of explaining Scientology's eight dynamics, the student is required to write down all their "Overts and Withholds." An Overt is any sin you did through your entire lifetime, and a Withhold is something you hold back or that you know someone else did. This book describes these as 'unethical' acts to pro-survival.

We were given gobs of clay to make tiny men and different scenes to demonstrate all eight dynamics. We labelled each object with tiny pieces of paper so the supervisor could read the demo scene easily.

Hubbard emphasises that:

> Dishonest conduct is non-survival. Anything is unreasonable or evil which brings about the destruction of individuals, groups, or inhibits the future of the race. The keeping of one's word, when it has been

sacredly pledged, is an act of survival, since one is then trusted, but only so long as he keeps his word. To the weak, to the cowardly, to the reprehensibly irrational, dishonesty and underhanded dealings, the harming of others and the blighting of their hopes seem to be the only way of conducting life.

When I read these words today, I see Hubbard's finger pointing back at himself and his 'Cult of Narconon.' In my opinion Scientology is dishonest, unreasonable, evil, destructive, weak, cowardly, and criminal to name a few. They lie because of their fear of consequences of the real truth and cowards in their own fear of self-destruction.

Perhaps the next part of Book 6 explains well *why* Narconon Trois-Rivières was shut down and destroyed itself from within?

Hubbard states:

The sexually promiscuous woman, the man who breaks faith with his friend, the covetous pervert are all dealing in such non-survival terms that degradation and unhappiness are part and parcel of their existence.

This "Covetous Pervert" quote by Hubbard reminded me of the movie *Silence of the Lambs* when Anthony Hopkins, playing the starring role of Hannibal Lecter says, "We begin by coveting what we see every day. Don't you feel eyes moving over your body, Clarice? And don't your eyes seek out the things you want?" Narconon staff violated Hubbard's own code of ethics in the highest degree. The lies, sexual predators, human rights abuses, and staff using drugs — all contradicted what the 'master' preached. They coveted.

And the gall of 'master' Hubbard to be writing such demands when he himself was the opposite including being married to two wives at the same time, is beyond belief!

I had already discussed my misdeeds with my Alcoholics Anonymous (AA), 'sponsor' many years ago and made amends as best I could, so going back over them again with people I didn't trust or like, was not my cup of tea.

But Hubbard was very crafty in writing his jargon — ever so subtly with gradients, convincing the student to fess up.

Hubbard writes, "By seeking to invoke his "individual right" to protect himself from an examination of his deeds, he reduces, just that much, the future of individual liberty for he himself is not free. Yet he infects others who are honest by using their rights to freedom to protect himself." So, I took this quote as telling me I wouldn't be free unless I allowed Narconon to examine my deeds and if I didn't write them out, I would be infecting others.

It took me a couple of days to think back a few decades and write down all my Overts and Withholds on a few pages of lined paper. Then I was told to hand them to the course supervisor who would then take them to the Case Supervisor.

Another Battle Begins

I told the supervisor, "There's no way I'm handing these in for someone to hold onto and read or make copies — this is very personal stuff!"

"But you have to David," he replied.

"I don't HAVE to do anything I don't want to do and I'm not giving them to you, period!" I replied.

I left the course room and went over to my room to rest and it wasn't long before security showed up telling me to go see Charles in Qual ... again.

I explained to Charles that I didn't want these handed in to be photocopied and spread around. He agreed to read them by himself and give them back to me when he was finished. So, I left him with it, not suspecting they would be copied. What a mistake!

I would learn later, after speaking out against Narconon, *why* they insisted the students write their most private misdeeds. Even though Narconon staff assured the students that their files were confidential, their moral and ethical code went out the door and down the crapper when attacked by any ex-Narconon student. Not only did they not keep my files confidential, but fabricated and manufactured unconscionable lies about me.

The more I spoke out, the more they attacked me at every turn, including turning others, including my own daughter against me.

L. Ron Hubbard wrote a policy 'attack the attacker' for the correct procedure for attacking enemies of Scientology.

The day I went back to retrieve my belonging from Narconon, I was declared an ENEMY on my Facebook wall by executive, Sue Chubbs.

Being an enemy of Scientology, I was 'Fair Game' and the 'Dead Agenting' began immediately. The 'Fair Game' policy meant I was a 'Suppressive Person' and "may be tricked, sued or lied to or destroyed." The 'Dead Agent' policy meant "start feeding lurid, blood, sex, crimes on the attackers to the press" or whoever else that would listen, resulting in my credibility be questioned.

In the days following my escape, executives told other staff that the reason I had left (blown), was because I had relapsed back into drug addiction. But, unbeknown to them, I was so distressed with diagnosed PTSD I ended up in the hospital emergency where blood tests proved I was drug free.

Other blatant lies were told to new staff that I belonged to a hate group called 'White Face' and was handing out pamphlets instructing people how to commit suicide. This was such a ridiculous and unbelievable claim, that Rob Piro wrote about it in his book after leaving Narconon *When God Called on My Cellphone*.[16] Not only will the student's confessions today be used tomorrow, but also anything they wish to invent or manufacture to cover their asses from their crimes and abuses ... This is Scientology policy.

Scientology could not change or alter Hubbard's 'Dead Agent' policies even if they wanted to — it's is a high crime to do so. Cynthia Kisser wrote something that rings true:

"Scientology is quite likely the most ruthless, the most classically terroristic, the most litigious and the most lucrative cult the country has ever seen. No cult extracts more money from its members." Indeed, ruthless, but on the verge of imminent collapse in the years to come perhaps?

Chapter 15

A Cult of Quackery and Confusion

I could not believe Narconon was telling us we could drink alcohol, but be careful not to drink too much or in excess! Nearly every recovering alcoholic will insist that one drink is too much and a thousand drinks are not enough when discussing their addiction. I have seen it time and time again that for a chronic alcoholic, taking that first drink is a recipe for disaster and death.

Of the entire eight Narconon books, Book 7, *Changing Conditions in Life Course*, was the most confusing of them all and forms part of the foundation of Scientology's greed, power, and control over members. Narconon production stats must be handed into head office every Thursday afternoon by 2 pm — without fail.

Narconon's Book 7 is where grooming and recruiting students for potential staff members begins. It's all about statistics and producing products, and as such, Narconon graduates are labelled as *products*.

In the Narconon course room for Book 7, students had clay demos spread out on the tables, demonstrating different products, such as making and selling hot dogs, books, bricks, you name it, the demos showed it.

This is played out in Scientology terms as, "The greatest good for the greatest number of dynamics," meaning that which is good for the Scientology group and their own survival. It's a selfish cult that is never seen feeding the homeless or poor. These people are looked upon as 'degraded beings' —

dead-beats, and the dregs of society. Scientology only seeks out those who are 'able' and "making the able more able." Staff who are unproductive or 'downstat' are told to 'get their ethics in'. Public members are told to call us when you have money and are able again. The opposite view should be true in a group that espouses to make the planet free.

The so-called 'Church of Scientology' and their front groups, is not about love, compassion, empathy, and more importantly, charity. This cult focuses on "making money, make more money, make other people produce as to make more money." — L. Ron Hubbard, Hubbard Communications Office Policy Letter, 9 March 1972.

The 12 'ethics conditions' in Scientology are Power, Power Change, Affluence, Normal Operation, Emergency, Danger, Nonexistence, Liability, Doubt, Enemy, Treason, and Confusion. Each dynamic is assigned a condition formula to work through by the students.

Being confused as hell from the get-go on page one, some of my condition formulas had me pegged as me being in 'confusion'. In the Narconon program we had to work our way up to 'Normal Operation', doing all kinds of crazy, bat-shit stuff to appease the supervisor and move on up to higher conditions of so-called "Survival." The theory in Scientology is that a person will always be in one of these conditions with regard to any area of life. And just because some of these formulas made no sense to the addict didn't matter. Because Hubbard wrote it, it must be right was the rule and staff dared not disobey to deter from his written words.

So, being in a condition of 'confusion', I had to 'Find out Where I Was' and then move on up to 'treason' where I had to "Find Out That You Are" was the real mind-twister of the entire circus show. I had absolutely no clue what the hell the command meant — not a clue!

When I asked the course supervisor what the phrase meant, he just repeated "find out that you are." I was so frustrated and angry I could barely contain myself from kicking him. Then we would know for sure exactly where I was at.

The supervisor was not allowed to give his opinion — no clues or any of his own thoughts or advice whatsoever. He could only point me back to the book text.

Course room supervisors were not viewed as, nor did they act as teachers.

A Cult of Quackery and Confusion

They only made sure we read the text and performed the written commands or directions. I had never in my life experienced such ridiculous and absurd nonsense. Now I understand why Rob Piro called Narconon "Nonsensenon" in his book — indeed, quite fitting.

Once I "found out that you are" I had to move up into the condition of Enemy, "Find out who you really are." Just reading some of this again — proof-reading before being published makes my head spin.

I was a good person who cared deeply for my children and friends — that's all that really mattered to me. I was happy to be drug free and able to make choices about my future. But little did I know that Scientology executives had plans for me far above my imagination — some that still affect me today.

One executive, Sue Chubbs, crossed the Scientology-Narconon line ... She was squirreling the Narconon program, going rogue.

She instructed the supervisor to have me view a video introduction to Scientology as part of my program. I was taken upstairs to the executive board room and watched the video while Chubbs looked on. After few questions, I returned to the course room.

But the head course room supervisor found out the next day and was livid. He was much higher up in the Scientology teachings than Chubbs, and couldn't understand *why* she would do such a stupid thing?

The Narconon program was NOT in any way whatsoever, to be seen as connected to Scientology and Sue Chubbs had blown it as far as he was concerned. He met with executives, insisting it never to happen again.

Scientology claimed that Narconon was a 'secular' program, not a 'religious' program as in the Church of Scientology. The video I was instructed to watch was taboo because it would connect the two entities as one.

After a few days dealing with 'confusion', 'treason', and 'enemy' conditions of my past, I began the long, drawn out 'DOUBT' condition formula. This one was far more complex and dealt with a person who "cannot make up one's mind as to an individual, a group, organization or project." Basically, I had to understand the bad drug user group I used to belong to, examine that group's statistics, and decide whether that group should be attacked, harmed, or helped.

Then I had to examine the new pro-survival group I was in now and do everything possible to help the group improve their statistics. Of course the real eye-opener was the next condition of 'LIABILITY' where I was instructed 'how to' increase the cult's statistics.

In 'liability' I proclaimed WHO my friends were, and most disturbing, I had to "deliver an effective blow to the enemies of the group one has been pretending to be part of despite personal danger." In other words, for me, I was instructed to write a scathing letter to a health agency damning the government's methadone program and praising Narconon as a drug rehab center.

The last step of 'liability' was going around with a clip board with a written summary, asking staff and students to allow me back into the 'pro-survival' group of Narconon by signing their name. It was kind of odd and somewhat embarrassing, but I was nearing the end of the program and just wanted it done.

The next four conditions of Nonexistence, Danger, Emergency, and finally Normal Operation, went well — a few more clay demos, and I was finished. Little did I know at the time, that these condition formulas were preparing me to be a staff member for Narconon?

Narconon Book 8 and the final process of cult indoctrination was *The Way to Happiness* philosophy of Hubbard. For me, it was one of the stupidest of all eight books. Besides instruction on keeping my body clean, brushing my teeth, and don't break the law, as well as other "thou shalt not" statements, I was STUNNED by Narconon's stand on drinking alcohol!

According to Book 8 it was OK to drink alcohol but not in excess. I had to write an essay about 'what is meant by do not take alcohol in excess' and 'give an example of the effects of drinking too much alcohol'.

I could not believe Narconon was telling us we could drink alcohol. Nearly every recovering alcoholic will insist that one drink is too much. I have seen it time and time again that for a chronic alcoholic, taking that first drink is a recipe for disaster and/or death.

And even for drug addicts, gulping booze more often than not, lowers inhibitions, and leads them back down the spiral of drug addiction.

I already knew that some Narconon graduates were drinking — I was given a glass of wine at the staff apartment complex when I arrived, and saw bottles of booze in the fridge. Now I understood why.

What Narconon was preaching and teaching was crazy, and for someone just finishing their drug rehab program, it sounded absurd, ridiculous, and dangerous.

After completing Book 8, some students were taken upstairs for a 'reach and withdraw' session with alcohol and drugs on the table in front of them. Real drugs! One student stated: "The last thing I wanted to see or touch before leaving Narconon, was more drugs." It was a process of being commanded to reach for the drugs, touch the drugs, and then withdraw the hand over and over again until there were no bad thoughts or feelings.

I refused to participate in the 'reach and withdraw' sessions but was subjected to a different wild and crazy routine of Hollywood acting that went on for two full days.

Near the end of my program, Narconon executives had convinced me to join staff as an Ethics Officer or Course Supervisor. I decided to take the supervisor's course to help students through their program.

But first I had to complete an "extended Narconon program" where I was directed to endure some 'Tone Scale' sessions of me acting out all the different levels on the scale. They said this would handle some issues the staff felt were affecting me and others negatively.

Staff saw me as a person who couldn't handle my emotions whenever I gave a short speech to students on Friday afternoons.

I knew what some students had suffered through in their past and when I stared out at the crowd of students, I had tears and trouble talking. I could feel other's pain and felt so sorry for what I knew the 'new-bees' would have to go through.

Or, if one of the young students told me their agonizing story recently, I would see them in the crowd and it was very hard to focus on what I wanted to say.

Other times I would reflect decades back or to times of torment at Narconon, and get very upset. It was horrible being on stage at times, but I knew I had to 'talk the talk' as expected from staff. I had to praise Narconon even if I was confused and felt something just didn't seem OK or right.

So, for two, long days, I sat on a chair with a Scientologist giving me commands to act out different 'tones'. "Just pretend you're an actor, David," one said.

Dante's Eighth Circle

I was told these 'tone scale' sessions would help me suppress my feelings and help me be able to talk to people without breaking down with emotions. The Case Supervisor, Marc Bernard, told me Narconon was "going to turn the marrow in my spine into solid bone." But for me, I really didn't want to be an asshole like Marc — I wanted me to be me. I was fine with WHO I was and how I interacted with others. "How dare they want me to pretend to be someone else," I thought.

No matter how loud or often I was commanded to act out certain 'tones' of 'hate', 'terror', 'dying', and 'total failure' on their cult tone scale range, it wasn't good enough for the staunch Scientologists. For two agonizing days I sat in the torture chair being worn down hour by hour.

I'm not sure who gave up first, the Scientologists or me, but after all was said and done, I felt no different — determined to just be me.

Chapter 16
All Was Well in Hell: Slave Labour and Drama

I reached into my staff mail box and pulled out my first piece of mail from someone and was stunned! "I am a porcupine, but when you turn me over I have the sweetest meat you will ever taste," was scrolled across the page.

Besides having no addiction counsellors or therapists to help us through our tough times — nothing else resembled a drug rehab treatment center.

Within a one month period, five of us were recruited onto staff as soon as we finished our program. I was taking the supervisors course, others trained to be ethics officers and word clearers and such.

Narconon was in upheaval at this time. There was a team of two from Narconon International in California, four from Narconon Canada, and Brad Melnychuk from ABLE Canada. Also, there was some from the church of Scientology in Montreal. ALL THERE AT THE SAME TIME!

Narconon Trois-Rivières had revenues in the millions and the sharks were circling for their chomps at the stock pile of money. Hundreds of thousands were sitting in Narconon's 'building fund' and money was being bled off up into the cult coffers.

With all these corporate entities and their Scientology staff working under one roof, the tension at times was as thick as flies on the Narconon kitchen flypaper strips.

Narconon Canada executives took over and removed the Trois-Rivières director, Marc Bernard from his post. Executive Aline Proulx, from Narconon

Canada, was appointed as the Establishment Officer (ESTO), and she ruled over all with a stern and manipulating fist. She had direct contact with Scientology's 'Office of Special Affairs' director, Yvette Shank, and Narconon International, California executives.

Although Narconon Trois-Rivières had raked in huge profits, some of the funds were apparently squandered where it should not have been. One of the executives had spent money on expensive media advertising to French Canada, and sponsored golf tournaments.

Proulx was appointed to her Narconon Trois-Rivières position of power by Scientology's hierarchy. She was appointed to oversee all divisions at Narconon and re-organize where needed.

Revenue income stats were crashing and more heads would roll. With the dip in funds, and fewer new student intakes, Proux moved staff around, hired new staff, and pressed staff to produce harder than ever. Friction between executives was evident, but nobody dared question Aline Proulx.

Financial corners were cut at every turn, including new graduates being hired and coerced into accepting a pittance of less than $100 per week for long, hard hours of stressful work.

As more funds were bled off, veteran staff in the kitchen and elsewhere did not receive their pay checks. Some weeks only a small advance on pay was given in cash. Eventually, valued staff, such as cooks, quit without notice, and students were pressed behind the kitchen counters and grills. Patients, who had paid $23,000 to be treated for their addiction, were now being exploited for free, slave labour!

So vampirish was this cult, that even I and the other four staff recruits didn't receive our mere $90 net pay for our week's work — only a few bucks in cash to tie us over till the next let-down. Some of us newbie staff had our rooms under the dorm wings and we ate at Narconon, paying up to $3.00 for each meal at times.

Cash was being squeezed from every person — Executives from ABLE and International were walking around checking out the delivery of Scientology processes on the students and at other times huddled in meetings.

My first day of working for Narconon was a head-spinning, jaw-dropper that I will never, ever forget. I reached into my staff mail box and pulled out my first piece of mail from someone and was stunned!

All Was Well in Hell: Slave Labour and Drama

The letter was a one-liner only with a signature 'Aline' on the bottom of the page.

"I am a porcupine, but when you turn me over I have the sweetest meat you will ever taste," was scrolled across the page.

"Is this why Aline had put her hand on my leg the other day? Is this why she was being so nice to me," I thought?

I took the letter down to my daughter's Ethics office, and she too, was stunned at the words. The other Ethics Officer was called in, but he, being the usual jerk-off he was, just laughed and said, "C'mon Dave, take one for the team." I showed the letter to a few other students who I trusted, and to the withdrawal specialist before going over to my daughter's apartment that evening.

Being in fear of Aline, nobody offered me advice about what to say or do about the sexually explicit letter. I had been at Narconon for six months as a student without any romancing and I certainly didn't want an affair with a Narconon Canada executive.

The next morning at Narconon, yelling was heard down the halls as Aline shouted at me, "Why the hell did you show my letter to people - do you know how embarrassing this is for me — I'm out of here for a few days to Ontario!" Apparently, Sue Chubbs went to Proulx's office and asked her what the hell she was doing by pressing me to have an affair?

Aline told me that she viewed Sue's comments as an intrusion into her personal affairs and told her:

"Unless you have any Narconon business to discuss with me, get the fuck out of my office right now!" Then raving mad, with travel bags in hand, she headed out the door for Ontario.

Some staff thought the entire ordeal was hilarious, but not me, I felt like I was being attacked by Aline, and laughed at by others. It was very humiliating.

I was feeling so stressed, I went over to see a staff member in withdrawal for an assist. After I lay down on the assist table, I heard: "Oh David, I'm a porcupine but when you turn me over I have the sweetest meat … " Even though I laughed, I replied "this is NOT funny — how would you like to be in my position having to deal with Aline?" So, here I was in Quebec with Narconon who drained all my finances - I couldn't speak French, and no

Dante's Eighth Circle

funds to travel back home to British Columbia thousands of miles away. I felt trapped like in a Zombie horror movie with darkness all around me.

A few days later, Aline was back in her office and a security officer directed me to go see her in her upstairs office. It was a small room with a desk, staff ethics file cabinet off to the side, and a single bed squeezed in near the window.

I sat across from her as she passed me a document for me to read. It was a "relationship" contract!

Several options were available for me concerning my relationship with Aline. One listed a '2D lover', one 'boss-staff', one 'sex but not committed', and a few others. I was shaking my head as I looked over the top of the paper at her, and then said, "I don't want, nor am I signing any contract agreement with you for a relationship — period," and passed the ridiculous document back to her.

Aline looked at me in a stern face and tore up the document, dropping it into the waste basket.

She then discussed about me having any job I wanted at Narconon, including being the executive director after a while. She said she controlled who went where and who obeyed who in the organization. "What do you want, David — you could be the director here in about 18 months." It was like she viewed me as a possession or toy that could be bought.

I was upset that she would even think of such a thing as a relationship contract — I had never heard of such a thing in the workplace. As I got up from my chair to leave, Aline walked around the desk and said, "Ok, can I at least have a hug before you go?" I said, "Sure, of course." Aline reached behind my neck and pulled me down towards her and gave me a kiss.

Shortly after I left her office, one of the Scientologists, Charles, who put me through the Tone Scale sessions, asked me if I wanted to get away for a while and go downtown for a coffee.

At the time, I never thought about this kind gesture, but then again, I didn't understand how devious or evil Scientology was, and that some members could be manipulating me for information. In this case, it appeared he was ordered to 'feel me out' and find out something that Aline didn't know and wanted to.

All Was Well in Hell: Slave Labour and Drama

It was mostly small talk about Narconon and staff as we drank our coffee and watched the interaction of people around the café. After being a student at Narconon for six months without any interaction with outsiders, I saw the colours people were wearing as extra bright and a faint memory of normalcy around me.

After some prodding, I told Charles that I did not want any relationship with Aline or anyone else, as a matter of fact.

"But David, you kissed her and now she's confused," Charles replied with a raised eyebrow. "You mean Aline kissed me, right Charles — it's not what you think," I replied.

"So, I was right, Charles was not being kind by taking me out for a coffee, he was on a mission ordered by Aline Proulx," I pondered.

We left a short while later and drove back to the compound in silence.

With good staff quitting, production spiralling down, Aline was under the thumb of Scientology powers up-lines and she was visibly distressed. Feeling so distressed, she was unable to leave her room one morning for breakfast.

Staff 'roll-calls' were intense. Narconon International staff would try to raise our tones by using their 'Chinese School' training on us. A lady stood at the front of our lines and shouted out some L. Ron Hubbard tech and we had to yell it back in unison as loud as we could. It was brainwashing loud!

At staff roll call one morning, Aline walked over to center stage and said with a stern face, "Ok, I want ALL of you to write up your OW's (overts and withholds) and hand them in by tomorrow morning." It was such a mess at the center and stats was dropping so fast that Aline or her superior decided there was a Suppressive Person amongst us and others were in a PTS condition that needed handling. She gave fair warning that everyone MUST start writing, or else.

One of the graduate students, and a dear friend, was taking courses to open their own Narconon in the Ontario area. It was her second time through Narconon and she also had a rental unit down the road at the staff apartment complex.

Aline was paranoid about this new Narconon being opened without her and Narconon Canada being in control over it. It was Narconon Canada's directive from International and ABLE, to see that all aspects of any new center be overseen by 'Canada' executives — especially by Aline and her sister who was also an executive of Narconon Canada for expansion. Of the two sisters, Aline was undoubtedly the more intelligent, and accordingly, Aline had kept her sister out of ethics trouble on more than one occasion.

Aline directed me and the new Ethics Officer in training, to go visit the new Narconon owner prospect at her apartment to feel out what she was up to. On the second day, I went by myself, but to me, nothing was really out of sorts. She was a really nice person, and only wanted to help suffering addicts.

The only thing that perked Aline's ears was the report from me that Narconon Canada would NOT be welcomed to visit the new center or give directives on how it would be operated.

I felt very uncomfortable spying on a friend and had the strangest dreams for many days — very disturbing and upsetting. It just seemed very wrong and not one does to a friend. But Aline insisted it was "for the greatest good of the group" and all would be fine in the end.

I asked Aline if this was the 'suppressive person' she was looking for, and she replied, "… yes it is, and I'll take it from here."

"What do you mean, is she a suppressive person or not and what are you going to do," I responded? This person, as far as I was concerned, had helped many people and didn't deserve any harm.

"Yes, David, she is a suppressive person, but she will remain an 'undeclared' SP … there's too much money involved if I rock the boat right now," she said calmly.

And Aline was right. Although the new Narconon in Ontario never did open as planned, forty new students were signed on in a negotiation at a slightly reduced package rate for the undeclared SP. Hundreds of thousands were involved, and Narconon in Trois-Rivières could increase their stats.

Later that same evening, my friend, the Ethics Officer in training and I were talking in our room about how crazy this entire secret stuff was and how it seemed like we were living in some kind of science fiction movie.

A few days later, he was moved into a house and shacked up with a Narconon staff member, and soon after, expecting a new baby. The pregnancy took him by surprise, but he seemed thrilled about it at the time. A group of us went over for a BBQ one evening and the new couple appeared happy and getting along well.

But it was not to be and his new girlfriend miscarried, losing the baby. My friend was upset for a few days, but appeared to me as being somewhat relieved that a forced responsibility was not pressing him anymore. I thought he would have made a great dad as long as he could remain free of addiction and not change from the caring person he was.

After I escaped Narconon, he would be pressed into writing a statement against me to the Quebec Human Rights Commission. It was a simple letter with no factual substance that I easily rebutted and I turned the focus around, and back to the abuses. It was his opinion only, and I knew where he was pressured from.

Not receiving our meager pay was taking a toll on all of us and I could see the stress level rise day by day. One of the new recruits came to me one morning and said he was leaving. He was the maintenance duty person and kept things fixed and running.

"David, I need to get another job where I'm paid — I can't keep doing this … " he said in a low tone. He was a great guy who hitch-hiked all the way to Narconon Trois-Rivières to get clean and sober and had many talents. As with so many other Narconon graduates, he was living with the 'Qualifications Officer' in one of the staff apartments down the road. It seemed there were more shack-ups between staff and graduate patients than one could keep track of.

"Ok, I feel the same as you and I'm going to look for another job too if they don't agree to pay us minimum wage — I'll go talk to Aline right now," I said.

After a very short meeting with Aline, I went back downstairs and told my friend that we would all now be paid at least minimum wage and we both agreed to tough it out for a while longer.

But even with minimum wage being promised, it really didn't matter. There were too many sticky fingers in the pie from 'NN International', 'NN Canada', and 'ABLE'. On paydays each week, we were promised this and that about our pay, but only received a small advance. The slaves were getting screwed … literally, and Scientology had billions in reserves.

Even if I wanted to leave and go home, it was impossible with no money to buy a ticket home. I was far beyond angry and frustrated!

students who paid tens of thousands to be treated for their addictions were working in the kitchen and keeping the center clean and liveable. Those who balked and disobeyed rules were kicked out and sent home or dropped at a homeless shelter. It was a *do-as-I-say* or *face-the-consequences* nightmare.

Frequently, when students were in trouble, the fault was not entirely their own. Staff weren't doing their jobs. All too often, they couldn't have, even if they tried, because they were too stoned or drunk. Many were hungover from the previous night's binge. One Registrar who relapsed was sent to the Alberta Narconon, and the senior Ethics Officer would soon be in the Narconon Trois-Rivières program again as a student.

It was bad … really bad.

I was sitting on the couch down at the apartment complex one evening when a phone call came in from Narconon. It was my daughter trying to convince her boyfriend, the senior Ethics Officer, to go down to the center to help her search a 'care package' for drugs. One of the other students had tipped off 'ethics' that drugs were coming in by way of being wrapped in a balloon and stuffed inside a shampoo bottle.

John was drinking that night and too drunk to drive or even speak without slurring his words, and said, "Go down to the kitchen and get a shrimp skewer and stick it down in the bottle to see if you feel anything … " and laughed out loud.

I knew that all the shampoo should have been poured out into something and examined for drugs, but talking to Mr. Know-It-All while he was drunk, was impossible. Most of the staff at Narconon were not trained to work at drug rehabs and especially, knew nothing about searching and finding smuggled drugs.

The cocaine in the shampoo bottle was missed in the haphazard search and it turned into a devastating relapse night at the center for more than one.

On another occasion, the drugs were hidden in the back of a pair of stereo speakers and no screwdriver was available to open the boxes. Again, the drugs slipped through and party time messed up untold numbers of students.

All Was Well in Hell: Slave Labour and Drama

Early one morning about two am or so, I received a phone call while I was at a staff apartment. One of the Narconon staff members had lost their car keys while bar-hopping downtown in Trois-Rivières with another staff member.

I was summoned to rescue them: "Please come down in a taxi to help find the keys," one said. I could tell they were drunk. They were slurring their words.

The taxi dropped me off near the corner where I was told to go. I looked around and couldn't see either of them. I was getting angrier by the minute. Then I went around a corner and there they were — sprawled out on the sidewalk, up against a wall. They both laughed when they saw me, but I was in no mood. I literally had to reach down and grab their hands to pull them up to stand.

After thirty minutes or so of listening to their blubbering, and looking for the keys, I gathered them into a taxi and we went back to the apartment. They bounced off the walls while going up the hallway stairs and were making a lot of noise.

It was chaos as I shut the door behind me with sounds of vomiting and cussing from another person yelling in the apartment.

I went into a room and fell asleep soon after the two passed out.

The next morning nobody was laughing — not even a smile from anyone in the apartment — they knew I was livid. I could not believe that Narconon executives were allowing these parties and relapses to continue without saying a word. Apparently the center had few drug test kits left and was saving them for the new student intakes, so rarely were the staff tested.

Even after I spoke to several executives and staff at a BBQ about the rampant drinking parties, nothing was done to discipline or help the relapsed staff. As long as the staff member was putting in an effort to produce stats on their post, "all was well in hell" and continued on status-quo.

The parties continued, staff messed up using drugs and drinking while other staff played 'drug counsellors' to the helpless addicts. And the executives didn't seem to know their ass from a hole in the ground ... most of the time turning a blind eye to troubles not affecting them directly.

Chapter 17

Working for an Alien Cult: False Success Rate

The 75 million year old story of a Galactic leader named Xenu, had me mesmerized and glued to my monitor. Billions of aliens were dropped around volcanoes and blown up with hydrogen bombs and I'm supposed to believe these little buggers are attached to me and polluting my soul?

The supervisor's course was easy and took me less than two weeks to complete while still helping out in the course room occasionally when needed. The course had nothing to do with drug rehab or how to help distressed students — only the Hubbard quack science and tech was studied and applied.

Aline was still harassing me at every turn to play her sex game and security was at her beck and call to send me to her office. Late one evening, a voice at my staff bedroom door instructed me to go see Aline right away.

I guess she heard me coming down the hallway to her office because as I approached the door it opened and I walked in. The lights were dim and she stood by the side of her desk in a black, shiny nighty. Without detailing the next hour or so, I left confused and felt sick as I walked back to my room. "Why did I give in to this predator," I thought.

Aline was a cunning lady, always with a battle plan to attain her own wants and sick needs. She approached me one afternoon with her planned trip to Ottawa with me and the Ethics Officer in training. She suggested we rent a car and blow Narconon for some fun times in an English city.

Dante's Eighth Circle

Her sister was there receiving auditing sessions and we could rent a couple rooms at a motel, she said. I thought it would be great to get away from the distress, see the sights, and renting two rooms sounded fine with me.

But when we arrived at her chosen motel, one room was for the Ethics Officer and Aline convinced me into her room for the night. I felt deceived and betrayed, and very uneasy as her advances increased that night and for the next few weeks.

I had so many distressful events swimming around in my mind every day, that I couldn't function well without first going for a walk or talking to someone I trusted. I couldn't focus on my training or job, and sleep was filled with nightmares.

"God, I wish I had money to get out of here and fly home," I thought.

Sunday, June 21, 2009, I received more very upsetting news that had me sitting over by myself at a picnic table sobbing. I felt a hand on my shoulder and a voice saying, "David, what's the matter ... what's the matter?"

"My daughter is gone — she left with her visitor friend from BC in her Jeep without telling anyone or even saying goodbye to me," I said.

I explained that John told me earlier that morning that he and my daughter had a fight after she and her BC friend were drinking at a bar. She left the apartment at about 2 am with her friend — driving back home to British Columbia. She was desperate, leaving thousands in appliances and belongings behind.

It was 'Father's Day' that morning and I was looking forward to spending some time with my daughter. I couldn't understand at the time, why she would do such a thing — just up and desert her Dad, the students who loved her, and the job she 'SAID' she cared about so much.

As usual with many things at the center, nothing made sense for days about why she had 'blown'.

My dear, trusted friend, sat with me at the table with her arm around my shoulder ... just being a friend ... showing me that she cared — listening to what I said.

There was nothing anyone could say to calm me down. I blamed the executives for not having control over the staff drug use and drinking. I was angry at my daughter for partying too much instead of dealing with her troubles or seeking help to sort them out.

Working for an Alien Cult: False Success Rate

"But who was I kidding," I thought, "Narconon doesn't have any staff for counselling!" Even though I cared about the students, I began to view the center as a human warehouse of suffering — a place like no other. A MAD HOUSE of insidious mind rape.

I tried to avoid being around Aline as much as possible and would eat my meals down at the student end of the dining room. They were much more fun to be around than a bunch of executive Scientologists and other staff. But it wasn't long before I was forced to eat with the staff, not the students.

"David, you can't sit with the students at meal times now, you need to sit with the staff," Aline said one morning. I didn't argue, it wouldn't have helped and I knew just to do what she demanded or I could be out on the street at her whim.

Working as a course supervisor was a demanding task and I took the students up the flights of stairs to Qual numerous times each day. But one day my ankle began to ache and swell up into a throbbing pain. A few hours later, I was sitting out at a picnic table unable to walk the rest of the way to my room.

The pain increased more each minute until I could not even stand.

The staff blamed it on me being PTS to my blown daughter, and said I needed to go for an assist. Reluctantly I agreed, but the pain only increased until I was taken to hospital emergency. "So much for Scientology tech," I thought.

I waited for seventeen long hours in the Quebec hospital emergency room. My friend Rob was kind enough to stay with me. Aline and her kin showed up with a take-out food order for me, but nothing for Rob! I didn't say anything, but was embarrassed that they didn't think about my friend.

After the doctor examined my ankle he said it was most likely tendonitis and to uses crutches with no weight on the injury. I left with a pair of crutches hobbled out of the hospital to the van for the ride back to Narconon.

So now, being a supervisor was out. No going up and down the stairs all day long. My option was being a 'Word Clearer', which I insisted I wanted nothing to do with — I didn't believe in such nonsense, and hated it.

The other option was being on post as the 'Graduate Officer' in an upstairs office. My 'Post' entailed contacting more than 700 students to see how they were doing and establish the Narconon Success Rate. The

Dante's Eighth Circle

Registrars were using this data to lure in new Raw Meat intakes. Many of the terms that Scientology uses like "raw meat" disgusted me.

As the Graduate Officer, the things I saw and read were absurd. I took a "Product Clearing Course" and training for "Valuable Final Product" (VFP). These only took a day or so to complete. I became a so-called certified counsellor in aftercare and relapse prevention. And, of course, calculating the Narconon success rate was a real eye-opener!

They lied! It was a fraud like non other I had ever seen.

Basically, my job consisted of preparing statistics about the students or "Products" and having the data ready to send up-lines to Scientology.

If the students I contacted had relapsed, they were not counted as a valuable product. They could not be expected to perform what we needed ... promoting Narconon.

Also, I had to convince the ex-students who were doing well to send a new intake to Narconon. We were to suggest that their life was saved by Narconon and that they now "owed" a debt to help Narconon.

I was instructed to spend less time on the suffering relapsed students because Narconon did not want too many to come back at one time — it would not look good. Plus, spending time on new intakes would generate the full program fee of $23,000 instead of relapses coming back at half price.

Discharging graduating students was an easy task. It took only an hour or so to process them and send them back to the same environment they came from. I knew some that needed a half-way house or a similar step to ensure a safe environment, but my words fell on deaf ears and were met with outlandish comments from my superiors.

After the student interview was finished, the graduate is driven to the Montreal airport and dropped off to catch a flight home. If airports didn't have bars — there would be no problem, but they have many. Some can't resist the tug to sit down for "just one or two drinks" before their flight. Dropped off and left alone in the airport, relapses were common before the student even arrives back home ... if they do.

Back in my office of lies — Narconon executives are well aware that the only way for a Narconon student to remain clean and sober, according to L. Ron Hubbard, is to enroll in the "NED Drug Rundown" — offered at the Church of Scientology.

Working for an Alien Cult: False Success Rate

Scientology's own words about the "NED Drug Rundown" say: "On this rundown, the harmful effects of drugs are erased and a person is freed from the compulsion or need to take drugs. This service handles drugs and the real reason a person started taking them in the first place."

"Addressing drugs with NED technology removes the barriers that prevent progress up THE BRIDGE levels. It is a vital step on your NED program." What these quotations imply is that the Narconon program does NOT erase the harmful effects of drugs, nor does it free a patient from the compulsion or need to take drugs!

As evidence documents prove, Narconon is nothing more than a recruitment center for the Church of Scientology. It exists to expand its cult practices into the secular community using Scientology coercion and exploitation of vulnerable, very ill people. Aftercare of patients is all but non-existent.

After contacting the graduates, it was an easy task to establish that the Narconon Trois-Rivières promoted success rate was False — a Lie — a Con — a Fraud. The numbers on my computer screen were printed so I could show some executives that we did not have a 76% success rate ... not a 70% success rate — it was closer to 40% and when relapsed staff was included in the numbers, Narconon's success rate was about 20%.

I printed off three copies and kept one in my personal files just in case I ever needed to prove these lies.

When I told my superior, Andre Ahern about the false stats, I was instructed to add the numbers of students I couldn't contact into the 'doing well' column. "I can't do that, it's an unknown plus or minus," I said.

I refused to participate in what I viewed as fraud. "Just use the global success rate then, David," said one executive. I refused! I thought, "just because you have a box of apples and most taste good doesn't mean they all do — some are sour, some rotten, and some have creepy crawlers inside." This Narconon was all of these ... a box of fraud and lies.

The next morning at roll call, Commander Aline said she need 'all hands' to bring in more new students and appointed me as a new Registrar. There was not enough money to pay staff and bills and Narconon needed money fast! More importantly, Aline was driven to increase stats that had to be submitted uplines next Thursday by 2 pm.

Being a Realtor and Sub-Mortgage Broker for more than six years, and combined with my other marketing and sales experience, made being a Registrar easy for me. In hindsight, I feel guilty and ashamed that I convinced new people into, or in some cases, back to, Narconon after they relapsed.

But on top of being on post as the graduate officer and registrar, I also took on a massive task of forming a new charitable Foundation. I wanted to raise funds for addicts who could not pay for treatment. Drafting the documents for Revenue Canada to form the registered charity was something I had done in the early 1990's and was straight forward. At least I thought it would be.

When I told Aline I was making a list of potential Foundation board members, I told her I would not consider Scientologists and Narconon staff that were Scientologists. I wanted people who cared about people first, not money.

Once the application was approved by Revenue Canada's charity commission, the plan was for me to fly out to the Alberta tar sands and oil fields, and other industrial parts of Canada. I would meet with executives of wealthy companies and unions for donations for the new Foundation.

I did an online search for a name to be registered and had a list of several that I submitted to my superior, Andre Ahern. He returned the list with the name 'The Golden Dawn' written at the top of my typed list. I Googled the strange name and the search returned astonishing results!

I learned The Golden Dawn is a 'magical cult order', with rituals at the center of contemporary traditions, such as Wicca and Thelema.

Andre Ahern wanted the Foundation name of a CULT! I couldn't believe it. It was a creepy feeling as I read more about the Golden Dawn.

I told Aline there was no way in hell I was going to name the Foundation this crazy 'Golden Dawn' name, and insisted once again that no Scientologists would be on the board of directors.

A day or so later, I was told that I was wearing too many hats, and that I couldn't work on the 'Foundation Project' at Narconon Trois-Rivières anymore. I was to do it on my own time, not Narconon's.

So, I continue on with being a Graduate Officer, Registrar, and work on the Foundation on my own time before and after work. Once the Foundation was approved by Revenue Canada, I could use the list of email addresses and other contact information of students and sponsors, Aline said. But for now, the Registrars were being pressured to bring in money and I had to turn my focus for a while.

One young man, who asked to come back after he relapsed, was strung out on high doses of Seroquel, an atypical antipsychotic approved for the treatment of schizophrenia and bipolar disorder. I was told that he would have to go to Narconon's medical detox first before being admitted to Narconon.

What? I was unaware that such a Narconon medical detox existed and asked the other Registrar what it was all about.

"We have a motel room set up with two staff who watches over the withdrawal," I was told. "A motel room," I responded?

"Yes, don't worry about it Dave, he'll be fine — just get him here and have his parents send the extra money as soon as possible," he replied.

But it wasn't OK or fine. When I visited the student once he was out and at Narconon, it was nothing but horror stories of being held captive with no nurse or doctor to help him.

I was livid, to say the least, and the 'motel' scam was never used again.

Chapter 18

My Dark Escape from a Cult of Paranoia

Everyday in the heat, rain and cold, I ran, alone in the woods ... in the hills near our home. There I felt the gentle touch of God. And I heard His whisper, you're stronger now. It's time to tell the truth of what happened. Tell your story to give someone hope. —Nikki Rosen

As I had some extra time on my hands, I thumbed through the $700 case of Scientology books that Narconon gave me to read. They were all bright-coloured and wrapped in shiny plastic. There was a closet full of cases of books — ready to be given to anyone they believed could be converted.

I was beginning to see more and more each day that Narconon was a dangerous cult ... a fraud, and the false success rate proved to me that I was being conned.

I was stunned to see that ALL of the Scientology content in these books was exactly the same as in the eight Narconon books. Word for word!

After my daughter 'blew' Narconon, she emailed me some names to Google about Narconon and Scientology and I found a whole lot more than I expected.

One evening while up in my office late at night, I Googled "escape scientology" and clicked on a link to a website owned by Bonnie Woods in England. The top of the page said: "Escape — helping families under Scientology stress. Escape was formed in 1992 for the purpose of helping, advising, counselling families and friends who have loved ones involved in Scientology."

"Well," I thought, "I don't have a family member in Scientology — my daughter is out, but surely I, still being trapped, would qualify for help," I thought.

I then clicked on a "help pages" link and began to read what services Bonnie offered, but saw nothing that pertained to me — a person who was in and desperately needed help getting out. With nothing to lose, I simply clicked on "contact us" and sent a brief request for help.

Within about an hour or so, I received an email from Bonnie Woods at my private email account. On Sunday, October 25, 2009, at 11:39 pm, Bonnie sends me a message of hope:

"I am waiting to hear from our contact in Canada who in turn is making enquiries about how they might be able to help. What is the city that is closest to you? Is the center far away from the nearest town? I don't know if you can access our website without being found out but if you can I wrote a book called 'Deceived' which is available to download. The appendix of the book has a history of Scientology that you might find helpful. How did you come to understand that you needed to leave?" Bonnie continues:

"I do understand how confusing it must be for you. I have read parts of your blog and I can see that you are determined to recover and after everything that you have been through I know you will find the strength to come through this part of your journey as well." I was in tears reading her response. It seemed incredible that someone cared and believed what I told had told her was true.

I had been coerced by the ESTO Officer, to move out of Narconon Trois-Rivières and live over at the new Narconon Canada house that had been set up with a small computer space for me. But I feared communicating from there, as any staff could easily walk up and see what I was doing.

I knew if any Narconon staff discovered I was leaving, I would be subject to immediate interrogation and an ethics cycle — something that I had previously experienced and feared. I planned to escape out of Narconon the same as my daughter did — without anyone being aware until after I was gone.

I still worked at the Narconon rehab center, but lived at Narconon Canada not very far away. I had my small offices set up at both places.

I replied to Bonnie the next day from my office at Narconon Trois-Rivières, on Monday, October 26, 2009 10:02 am:

"I am mid-way between Montreal and Quebec City, in a place called Trois-Rivières. It is a small city of about 80–90 thousand people. Over 90% are French speaking. I began to do some research on Scientology, (after seeing some strange things here), and became convinced this place is not what it is made out to be. All of the upper staff are Scientologists and the control over us is fierce and suppressive. Gosh, my language has been changed and brainwashed into speaking and writing the new words they've taught me."

"Anytime I've had a little cold or pain, I get interrogated in a PTS interview. Anytime someone wants to leave, they get torn down and labelled a person in TREASON. Just two minutes ago, someone came into my office to see what I was typing. They check my other emails. This I know for sure. This is not easy to live or function with. They are four paydays behind. The money they bring in just disappears. The ONLY reason I stayed here so long was to help the new people coming in. This is another reason that it is hard for me to leave." While waiting for a reply from Bonnie, I did a Google search that my daughter told me to do of Jean Paul Dubreuil who is an ex-Scientologist and the ex-husband of Narconon Trois-Rivières executive, Therese Sansfacon and father to other staff at Narconon.

Jean-Paul Dubreuil described how Scientology tore apart his marriage, disconnected him from his children and grandchildren, and ruined all of his dreams. More importantly, what exposed me to the real truth about the cult I was in were the Google results during my search — all thanks to my daughter.

The next search from my tiny upstairs office showed me the truth about all the lies that I had been duped into believing for so long. It was a shocker above shockers!

A video by "CBC TV — Radio Canada, a Narconon Expose by Emilie Dubreuil," produced on April 2, 2008, was a jaw-dropper for me. Here I was sitting in my Graduate Officer's office, with other staff only thin walls away.

I was watching and listening to an investigative report on the sacred secrets of Scientology's OT-III religious doctrines about space aliens and murder.

"OMG, I thought," as I was watching, "I hope these walls don't have ears right now or I'm toast!" I turned the volume down and read the English sub-titles as it played for nearly 18 long minutes.

It was an incredible video — It was a video about a 75 million year ago Galactic Alien leader named Xenu. I was mesmerized and glued to my monitor. The video claimed, billions of aliens were brought to earth and executed by dropping them around volcanoes. The aliens were then blown up with hydrogen bombs... And I'm supposed to believe these little buggers are attached to me and polluting my soul?

"I was conned, betrayed, and here I am in the middle of nowhere after being indoctrinated into the cult of Scientology," I mumbled in confusion. My head was kind of sore and spaced out after reading, watching, and listening to this 'way-out to lunch' stuff.

I didn't sleep for the next two days and when I did collapse in exhaustion, my nightmares were the most vivid ever — a scary and disturbing experience, waking up soaking wet several times.

It seemed like forever waiting until Bonnie contacted me again. My mind was hamster-spinning, stress was overwhelming and sleep escaped me. The time I had taken off from Narconon for a few hours to be by myself at the strip mall, was fresh in my thoughts. And now, I needed to get away again to clear my head and think.

I looked around the mall food court for Chinese food — I really wanted something to feel good about, and I loved Chinese.

But within an hour after leaving, my cell buzzed with text messages, "Where are you, we can't find you — call back right now," was demanded. I just ignored the intrusion. Living, eating and working at the cult compound 24/7, for long hours each day, had taken a toll and I needed some space.

But little did I know, a search party was on the prowl to find me and before I finished eating, the ESTO Officer was standing over me with quite the angry face. After some small talk, I was in the Narconon van and on my way back to hell.

As I waited for Bonnie, captive thoughts were spinning my head into distress and anxiety.

Finally! The next morning: Tuesday, October 27, 2009, at 8:54 am, I received the following message:

"HI David, thank you for explaining what has happened to you. It makes me feel very sad to know that your genuine desire and need for help ended in such deception and suppression. I can understand your desire to try and protect the new people coming in but I believe the only truly effective way to do that is to expose the conditions there."

"As you know we have friends in Canada who we trust. They have extensive personal experience with Scientology. They have some questions and immediate suggestions for you. I have written them below and I will let them know your responses as soon as I receive them. Do you need physical help to get away?"

"Can you be called directly on your cell phone number? You should get away as quickly as possible. It is utterly unreasonable for you to have to give notice and subject yourself to anymore pressure. Do not trust the people running Narconon and do not allow them to handle you."

"Do you have a place to go — any family? Can you provide the contact information for your friend in Montreal? If the immediate danger becomes too great you should leave the property and dial 911 and ask the police for help and to accompany you to retrieve your belongings."

"Are you concerned about what you have told Narconon staff or information they have about you?"

"Do you want the kind of protection you'd get from going to the media? Our friends have contacts in Quebec and even Trois-Rivières who have covered Narconon and could perhaps be helpful. Your circumstances and conditions at Narconon Canada deserve exposure."

"You have what it takes to walk out that door."

"Go with God"

"I know you have to find a safe time to answer all of this. I will send the answers to them as soon as you can let me know. It must be very difficult to think clearly. We'll keep praying as I know you are. Bonnie." I was so terribly distressed and overwhelmed, sitting in my graduate/registrar office with tears running down my face as I read Bonnie's email. I was relieved, angry, happy — so many emotions and not knowing or understanding why? All that mattered at that moment, was I had found someone who didn't know me, but understood my confused feelings.

Less than an hour later, I replied:

Dante's Eighth Circle

"Hi Bonnie — Thank you very much. Plain and simple, I am in some fear. So much at times, I have trouble breathing. I think it's just from the oppressive stress that is thrown at me every day. To be honest, I'm too nervous to answer all of your questions in writing on this computer in my office at Narconon Trois-Rivières. Can you imagine that? There is a lot more to this than you could ever think possible. Yes, you can call me on my cell: 819-701-1559. If I can't talk, I'll just say that you have the wrong number. Usually, from 12:30 to 1:00 pm is good. I can walk around the parking lot and they don't bother me." Bonnie replied: "Hi David, I understand how you are feeling. I have passed your number to our friends in Canada and asked if someone can call you. I'll let you know when I hear back from them. Stay safe. Bonnie." Bonnie mentioned the name 'Gerry Armstrong' as her contact in Canada, so I went to my friend, Google, and countless websites returned volumes of information about a man who had gone through hell after leaving Scientology in California. Lawsuits, threats, dead agenting, fair game — you name it, Gerry Armstrong endured it all.

I was happy to have someone helping me with as much experience as Gerry, but quite honestly, after reading what the cult did to him after leaving, I was stressed more than ever. I knew I had to be careful and cover all bases in my escape plan.

I did have a contact in Montreal who worked for the Canada Federal government and they offered to help by driving to Trois-Rivières and pick me up when it was safe — after dark preferably.

After I spoke to Gerry, Bonnie sent another email. Tuesday, October 27, 2009, at 11:38 pm:

"Hi David, I am very glad to hear that you have spoken to Gerry. I have received your last three messages but thought I would reply to them all on this one. I have forwarded them to Gerry just in case you only have time to write to one of us. Please do be careful not to put yourself in any danger while you are trying to document things. Your safety and well-being are the most important things right now. Do you have any timeframe in mind for when you want to leave? As always, stay safe — Bonnie." Frantic, I knew it was crucial for me to gather all my diarized notes and countless pages I had written over the past 11 months as a student and staff member. Some of the documents that Narconon had given me to use, in a now private project of creating and registering a new charitable Foundation, I packed away.

These documents were proof of the fraudulent success rate scam. Executives had harassed me to participate in this conspiracy to defraud the public and nobody would believe me unless I could provide documented evidence.

I had no idea when I would escape, or where I was going, but being prepared was a priority. Emails that I had received internally from executives and staff, I forwarded away to an outside private account, including many scanned documents that could substantiate the human rights abuses. Once forwarded to my private account, I forwarded these again to another more secure account.

I was anxious and becoming extremely stressed as I secretly packed away what I would leave with. I decided to leave most of my belongings, including my computer and personal items — only having a small travel bag filled with a few clothes and two large garbage bags filled with documents. Just writing of these past traumatic events, brings back unwanted, frightful emotions.

The next day, Wednesday, October 28, 2009, at 8:44 am, I sent a message to Bonnie, telling her I was leaving today:

"Please have Gerry contact me as soon as possible. I want to leave today somehow. There is another staff member leaving … at least one and I just can't stay here anymore. I want to expose what's going on here to the students before I leave, but I don't know if I should. They and many of their parents know me and trust me and will protect me if there is any trouble. If there is any Media available, 'this is the day'. I am a near basket-case, as far as my stress is right now. I look forward to hearing from you soon." A few hours later, Wednesday, October 28, 2009 at 2:02 pm, Bonnie writes back:

"Hi David, I have sent your message to Gerry. Probably best to leave as quietly as possible although I understand your desire to help them. I also sent your last message to Gerry and asked for help in finding somewhere to go, but I haven't heard back from him yet." I was working with two relapsed Narconon students at the time. One I knew well and was trying to help prevent his suicide. Even though I knew Narconon was not a good rehab, this person had sent me a long email, begging me for help before he died. I knew Narconon was a scam, but I wanted to help get him off the street, even if it meant Narconon temporarily until a safer rehab was found.

I was on my cell phone much of the day and used the new student intake calls as a 'ruse' to call my Montreal contact to pick me up near Narconon Canada after dark. I knew Aline would be at her hairdresser's appointment, covering up the dreaded gray, and once the colour was on her head processing, I had a short window to escape without being noticed.

Gerry Armstrong had contacted an investigative reporter, Émilie Dubreuil. She was with CBC TV — Radio Canada in Montreal.

Ironically, that was the video I had watched with the English subtitles that showed me how and why Narconon was 100% cult of Scientology. I contacted her by email and sent details of what was going on inside Narconon and why I was leaving. Emilie asked all the right questions and I answered in detail. I agreed to phone her when I was safe in Montreal.

On the evening of October 28, 2009, I was picked up and whisked away to a secluded Motel in Montreal and hid away for three days. Within an hour of being picked up, my cell phone began to ring and text messages poured in from Narconon staff, demanding that I immediately return and "face the music" for blowing.

One message spelled out that I would need to sit down with an executive and perform an ethics cycle, which would also include doing a "Condition Formula" of "Doubt", asking the "Group" to allow me back in.

The messages were aggressive and threatening in nature and caused me extreme upset and stress. But there was absolutely no way in hell I was going back or answering their questions. I had most of the answers I needed, and going back would only benefit them, not me.

After staying in the tiny Motel room, I moved to another location just outside Montreal where I could set up a secure computer connection, and contacted the reporter, Émilie Dubreuil.

I eventually met with the reporter on November 3, 2009. We decided to travel to Narconon in two vehicles. The reporter and TV crew in one — and me in another car with a friend.

I wanted to retrieve my computer, personal belongings, and the wages they owed me and return their cell phone. Sitting in the passenger side of my friend's small car, I scribbled my resignation on a sheet of paper and took photos of it.

My Dark Escape from a Cult of Paranoia

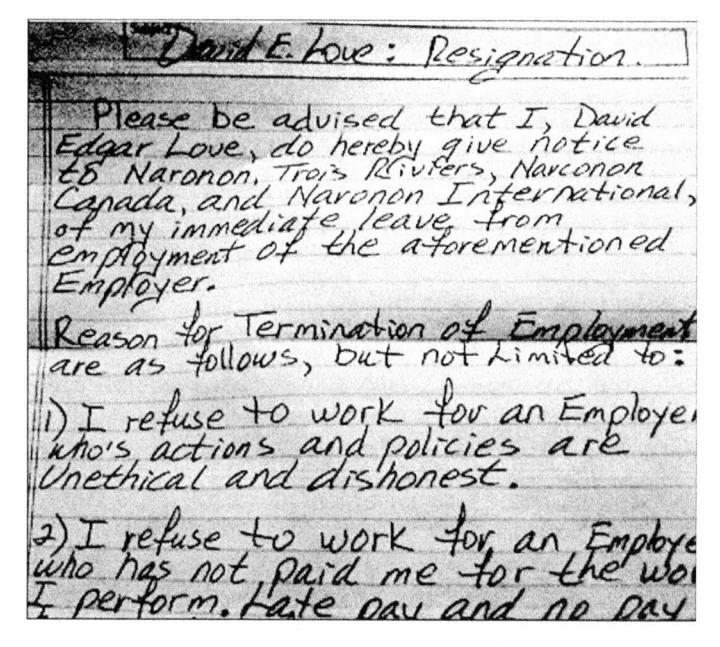

> **David E. Love : Resignation.**
>
> Please be advised that I, David Edgar Love, do hereby give notice to Naronon, Trois Rivières, Narconon Canada, and Narconon International, of my immediate leave from employment of the aforementioned Employer.
>
> Reason for Termination of Employment are as follows, but not Limited to:
>
> 1) I refuse to work for an Employer who's actions and policies are Unethical and dishonest.
>
> 2) I refuse to work for an Employer who has not paid me for the work I perform. Late pay and no pay

I phoned, and arranged for the local Police to escort me into the Narconon building. The CBC TV camera was up against the "Narconon Reception" window filming as the director, Marc Bernard, handed me my check. I handed Marc the phone and my resignation. The Police were inside with me and all was peaceful, except for my pounding heart and disoriented mind. Being back inside the center was strange — kind of surreal.

But I still needed to pick up my belongings over at the Narconon Canada office a few miles away, so the Police drove over to keep the peace.

Aline was there, as expected, with some other staff. She demanded I pay her about $300 or so for clothes she recently purchased for me with a credit card. I agreed and went to the bank to cash the check I just received and handed her the cash when I returned.

Knife cutting tension filled the air as I carried out boxes into the small car. Then just as I finished loading up the car with my stuff, the almighty Aline commented to me:

"David, PLEASE don't hurt Narconon, it wouldn't be right." I didn't look or reply — just got in the car and we drove away. What a relief. Looking back over my shoulder I saw the Narconon 'supreme ruler' standing in the driveway with a very low-tone face in apathy. Finally, I could breathe easier

Dante's Eighth Circle

… not concerned about being hounded down like a stray dog every time Aline didn't know where I was.

But was I really free? At that time, I wasn't really aware of how me 'Blowing' (leaving the cult) would affect so many people, including Aline who left Narconon in disgrace, 'Thrown Under a Bus' as it was called when Scientology fries somebody when they make huge mistakes as Aline had done.

She was one of the executive directors of the entity, 'Narconon Canada' who had violated L. Ron Hubbard doctrine and policy. She knew, or should have known, that having a 2D relationship with someone who was not friendly or open-minded to Scientology, was a "High Crime" and would not go unpunished.

The powers over Aline forced Narconon Canada to "Dissolve and Liquidate" on 2010-09-02 — with Aline moving to Ontario in seclusion. This was HUGE — Narconon Canada was the Scientology 'expansion' entity in Canada directed to open more Narconons across the country.

Somewhere in our drive over to Narconon Canada, we lost the CBC TV reporter, so we drove back to Narconon Trois-Rivières to see if she was there. As we neared the compound, I could see a parked Police car and Emilie interviewing Andre Ahern on camera. I got out of the car and took a few photos from the roadside and then we turned around and left for Montreal.

As soon as I arrived in Montreal, I looked on my Facebook wall and read a post by Narconon executive director, Sue Chubbs, declaring me an "ENEMY" of Narconon. I was now vulnerable to Scientology's "Fair Game" policy and may be "deprived of property or injured by any means by any Scientologist without any discipline of the Scientologist. May be tricked, sued or lied to or destroyed." A few days later, Emilie contacted me and I met her in a Montreal park with a large plastic tub filled with the new Scientology and Hubbard Dianetics books and tapes that Narconon gave me when I graduated the program.

The cameraman filmed all the material as Emilie interviewed me. She also had a reporter in Ontario interviewing two other ex-Narconon victims to confirm and verify the incredible story I told her about patient negligence and abuse.

"Finally," I thought after all the filming and interviews were done — "now the truth will be exposed about the dangers and abuse at Narconon." But it was not to be. When Emilie returned to CBC TV — Radio Canada to review all the footage from Quebec and Ontario, the Ontario tapes were missing — gone!

She explained nothing like that had ever happened before to her, and had no idea or proof of where the tapes were or disappeared to. Of course we had our own suspicions, but without proof, no allegations were made or expressed and the Narconon expose show was never aired.

Emilie would later write for a prominent newspaper in Montreal and travel with me to Senator Céline Hervieux-Payette's office on Parliament Hill in Ottawa for my second meeting in the Senator's office.

Chapter 19
Help from Anonymous

> We are Anonymous — Knowledge is free — We do not forget — Keep calm and expect us ...

After escaping Narconon, I was alone in a Motel hideaway for a few days before moving into a house and set up online with a secure internet connection. I continued to feel the stress and trauma from being at Narconon. Horrible nightmares were constant and exhaustion from lack of sleep wore me down.

I had never heard of Anonymous before — especially living in the cult compound where Narconon had many websites blocked, including Facebook and such. When I joined staff, I could access whatever I wanted, but, I was being monitored when I was on Facebook, and suspected that all websites I visited were visible to peering eyes.

Now that I was 'OUT' — I could surf the internet without concern or fear ... I was free.

While Googling around one evening, I came across a *Why We Protest* website and a thread named 'Narconon Trois-Rivières in Trouble' posted on August 8, 2009, by a person using the name Peterstorm. He was a member of the Anonymous Collective.

I remembered I had discussed this thread "topic" with an executive at Narconon. A new bill was proposed by the Parliament to apply mandatory certification for drug rehab centers in the province of Quebec!

I knew that this new legislation only concerned residential treatment centers in Quebec and being a Realtor for six years in land development and subdivisions, I was well versed in contract law. I felt there was a solution to bypass the new regulations. If Narconon tried hard enough and used available loop-holes to circumvent the new drug rehab legislation in Quebec, they had a possibility of staying open.

I thank God, that before I had time to discuss details with the executives, I escaped and didn't reveal what I knew. Actually, there were two loop-holes, but the law firm representing Narconon missed them both. I found it strange they could miss such a thing.

Peterstorm became a trusted contact and friend — helping me with media and visits at government agencies. He could read and speak French perfect and met with me to visit the Quebec Ministry of Health and Social Services in Trois-Rivières. While there, CBC TV — Radio Canada showed up to interview myself and the health ministry.

I was concerned that the Ministry did not have all the loop-holes covered, and showed them a quick sketch of how Narconon Trois-Rivières could stay open if Narconon discovered the flaw in the new legislation.

It would have been an inexpensive and simple manoeuvre for Scientology to keep their prized, 100 bed center open. But, Narconon insisted on filling Health Ministry files with success stories, propaganda and such, as opposed to directly addressing the legislation itself.

After I scribbled a sketch for the health agency official, he agreed it was loop-hole that could be exploited if Narconon recognized it, but "hopefully they wouldn't," he said. And if they did find the loop-hole, the Health agency assured me it could be closed. To this very day, they probably still don't know how they blew their potential chance to stay open ... at least for a while.

Then we were off to a newspaper interview for an hour or so before I returned to Montreal. The TV show aired that night with devastating effects. The reporter leaked documents from the Quebec College of Physicians against Dr. Pierre Labonte, the Narconon Medical Manager. Anonymous is expert at digging up and leaking insider documents.

As soon as I arrived back on my computer, I contacted Peterstorm about the meeting and decided what I should do next. I was pretty stressed and my mind was spinning while trying to process all the information.

At the end of November 2009, I received an email from a friend still on staff at Narconon and she was very upset. This person was my friend and she was loved by many of the Narconon students as a caring person — one filled with compassion that went the extra mile to help. She was kind to everyone — a real gem.

She expressed her concerns of being close to some staff who were not Scientologists and that they were being treated like slaves.

Narconon stated: "If you DARE speak out, you are fired immediately," she said.

The Narconon executives were harassing her — threatening to fire her if she contacted me. On Sunday, December 13, 2009 at 1:33 pm, she wrote:

"When they found out we were communicating ... he wanted me to enter my address and my password on his computer, but I didn't have my password. Even Thérèse Sansfaçon and Marc wanted me to write to you to say that I wanted nothing more to do with you — fat chance of that!! They aren't going to be telling me who I can communicate with." Many of the staff and students at Narconon wondered why I left and Executives were quick to answer with lies. One friend sent me an email from Narconon on Sunday, December 13, 2009 at 11:17 am:

"They are saying that you have back slid and that you have had a drug problem for 45 years. First of all, I don't believe that. Marc is the one that sat there and looked me in the eye and said that," the sender wrote.

I wasn't too concerned over what Marc Bernard was spouting off — many expressed their disproval of his character and credibility issues. In my opinion, Marc was just a glaze-eyed, cult worshipper who didn't know his ass from a hole in the ground. His way or the highway was his method of control and power over others. I never did like him, nor did he like me I suspect. What I was doing to expose Narconon to the media and government agencies was, without a doubt, causing him much grief and distress.

Then early one morning, my computer crashed and strange icons appeared on my desktop. I couldn't load programs and my screen froze solid!

I contacted another Montreal Anonymous friend and they helped me download and install Malwarebytes, an anti-malware program. Once downloaded, I had to install in 'Safe-Mode', and 'Run' it.

Walls of Trojan horse, Keystroke Logger, and Worm files appeared on the scan 'results' screen. Access to my computer files showed the dates between: October 28, 2009, and when I picked my computer up on November 3, 2009, including the files that were accessed between those dates.

"Welcome to the church of fear and paranoia," I thought. And I was one pissed off Irishman! "How dare they hack and violate me this way!" The Viruses appeared to be installed while my computer was in their possession before I went back to pick it up at Narconon. Once I quarantined all the viruses, my computer worked fine, but I soon replaced it with a new, clean laptop with beefed-up security.

Even though the cult may have seen some of the files I was working on, I had not gone to the website where there was important and sensitive, scanned documents stored online. Some I stored in an off-shore email account in Panama, and some at a storage account in Switzerland.

I then backed-up all my files and copied them to external hard drives that I stored in a locker. I gave my password to one Anonymous member just in case I should meet an untimely demise. I wanted ALL the documents, photos, and video published online as soon as possible if something happened to me.

Anonymous members from around the globe continued to help me with research and finding documents. Just knowing that I was not alone was a big help as I pressed on. This is a group of people who have relentlessly protested in front of Scientology organizations, and educate the public, media, and authorities.

For obvious reasons, and ongoing lawsuits I filed against Narconon and Scientology in Montreal, I dare not post more details of my connection with Anonymous. Suffice to say that all of the Anonymous people I dealt with, did everything legal, never crossing the line into illegal activity. What impressed me the most about Anonymous was that most of them had never been a member of Scientology. What motivated them to protest and picket Scientology's Narconon ? Quite simply, they cared about people. They refused to allow this powerful cult to commit fraud, tear families apart, and violate human rights and freedoms.

We had a common goal, and I am so very grateful for all their help.

Chapter 20

Legal Battles and Educating the Community

For there is but one essential justice which cements society, and one law which establishes this justice. This law is right reason, which is the true rule of all commandments and prohibitions. Whoever neglects this law, whether written or unwritten, is necessarily unjust and wicked. —Marcus Tullius Cicero

With a couple of days of online job searches, I had a job at a marketing company and moved into my own apartment within weeks. It was a grungy old apartment building in a rundown area of Lachine, on the outskirts of Montreal, but it served my purpose ... and still does today. I felt lucky because the previous tenant, who moved out of the bachelor pad, left their furniture. The land lord said I could have it all, including a small desk, hideaway bed, and kitchen table and chairs. There was even an old twenty inch TV that still works today.

My next chore was writing the formal complaints to the Worker's Compensation Board (CSST), Canada Competition Bureau, Quebec Labour Relations Board, Quebec College of Physicians, Ministry of Health and Social Services, and most importantly, the Quebec Human Rights Commission. I delivered documents in person to the Montreal office of the Canada Competition Bureau concerning Narconon's fraudulent success rate, and the agent photo copied everything for investigation.

Once the volumes of cover pages and supporting documents were submitted, I went for interviews at the government agencies. It was an experience I will never forget — indeed, a very stressful time. My first appointment was with a lawyer from the Labour Relations Board.

He was a strapping big man for a lawyer — kind of rough around the edges, but he knew Quebec Labour laws inside out. This case was for 'Psychological Harassment' that I was subjected to while being a graduate officer and registrar at Narconon. But this lawyer knew nothing about Scientology and I had to take him on a story journey step by step, pulling out evidence documents when needed to help him understand.

We eventually compiled a strong case and Narconon received a copy of the statement of claim with a time limit to respond. The Labour Board sent investigators to interview the respondents and witnesses and one was notably distressed, according to the lawyer — in tears during the interview.

My immediate superior, Andre Ahern, was apparently so stressed after I blew, that he was off work for quite some time. Narconon Canada dissolved soon after I blew and the executives were out of work, wondering what was coming next. I advised Narconon's law firm, Heenan & Blaike that I would use every available legal avenue possible to seek justice, and would not stop until the gavel of guilt slammed down loud.

In turn, Narconon's law firm sent me a strong letter, advising they would take swift legal action against me if I continued to 'tarnish' their client's reputation. They insinuated my Narconon patient records would be used to question my credibility. It was like a threat, extortion or black mail in my view and I responded with a counter-attack, stating Narconon executives and staff should be far more worried about their credibility than I should be. We had many letters back and forth, including thousands of pages I sent them.

I even filed a formal complaint to the Quebec Bar against Heenan & Blaikie for being in a 'conflict of interest' situation and that the law firm must recuse themselves from representing Narconon et al. There was a brief investigation and the Bar decided there wasn't quite enough evidence, but left the case open for me to appeal at a later date with more evidence.

One more case before the Labour Relations Board was for unpaid wages due. Narconon fought, saying I had agreed to receive a lower pay while being trained, but in Quebec, this is illegal and Narconon knew it.

I received a letter from their law firm offering to pay me the $2,555 owed if I signed their "Release and Discharge" document. It was a GAG order for me to stop talking to media and forbid me to talk or write anything critical about Narconon or Scientology. For each time I violated the agreement, I would have to pay their client $5,000!

I was having trouble making ends meet with my low paying job and didn't have enough money for rent, utilities, and food. I played along with the law firm a bit and stalled for time, not knowing what to do?

Anonymous put me in contact with a lawyer who knew all about Scientology and I sent them a copy of the Release and Discharge.

"David, do NOT sign this document," was the immediate reply. We spent the next several hours on the phone and exchanged emails in the early hours until I received a suggested 'revised version' by email. This was a document that would be for the benefit of me, not the cult. Narconon's lawyer was driving the hour and a half trip from Trois-Rivières to Montreal the next day to meet me in their Montreal office.

I arrived at their office the next day and already knew in my mind what the lawyer's reaction would be. We sat down in a beautiful board room with a long, shiny table and he opened his file, flashing a certified check off to the side as he laid the Release and Discharge in front of me. I was broke, only change in my pocket. I knew if I signed, I could be home in British Columbia within days — back with my family.

"Oh God be with me," I mumbled to myself as I pulled out the revised document and said. "Sorry, but I'm not signing that document, but here is one that you can have your client sign."

"What, I drove all this way and you're not going to sign the release I brought — why didn't you phone or inform me before I came all the way here," he said in anger and disappointment.

I replied, "Well, I didn't know for sure if I was going to do it my way until after you had left Trois-Rivières on your way here — in fact I didn't know for sure until a few minutes ago."

"My client will not sign that," he said.

I calmly said, "Well, that's not my problem whether your client will sign it or not, they're your client and your problem, so please deliver it to them."

Dante's Eighth Circle

He put the certified check back in the folder and closed it. Not a lot of money for most people, but to me at that time, it was a lot.

I stood up and walked out of the room, shaken somewhat from standing my ground with this arrogant cult representative.

It didn't really hit me until I was standing on the sidewalk beside the massive law office of Heenan & Blaikie — a law firm that boasted 500 lawyers in offices around the globe.

I remember saying to myself, "What am I going to do now, I'm up against these monster people and I'm broke ... I have no money to even buy groceries right now." I was in a daze.

I had enough change to buy some spaghetti noodles on my way home and started the water boiling on the stove while I turned on my computer to check my emails and browse the Anonymous forums for recent posts.

There was a few emails, but one that stood out was something called 'PayPal'. I had never seen or used this before and had no idea what it was until I clicked on it.

In peach coloured text, the email message said: "Guardian Angel (not real name), has sent you money," with a very kind note attached. For about thirty seconds I didn't understand or know what it was or meant? I just sat there staring at the screen ... not really thinking it was real.

Then tears poured down my face — I was overwhelmed with so many feelings of gratefulness and relief. The deep, beautiful emotions of being blessed by someone I had never met were incredible. I didn't even know who this person was. This person was thanking me in the email and I didn't yet understand why? It took a few days to transfer the funds from PayPal into my bank account and I was able to pay bills and buy food.

It made sense to me that I shouldn't have to sign Narconon's GAG order just to receive the wages they legally owed me and I expressed this in another email to their law firm.

On 'Good Friday', 2010, Marc Bernard, Narconon's executive director, along with Sylvain Fournier, the ex-Narconon director, met me in a café with a check in hand and my Tax documents I requested. A friend came to the meeting with me and placed a recorder on the table and turned it on. Marc Bernard signed the revised release document I provided and handed me a check for $2,555.

Near the end of the meeting, Marc asked me what would be a comfortable settlement to make all the rest of the complaints go away. I asked him if he was authorized to offer a settlement and he said he was authorized to hear my proposal and take it from there.

After dealing with these slippery and stall tactics Scientologists, and their ignorant lawyers for many months, I really didn't take Marc's question seriously. We exchanged a few words about me going back home and such, then I stood up and said with a smile "just add a couple of zeroes to this and we're done." Marc replied, "Ok, I'll take the offer under consideration," or something along those lines, and my friend and I walked out. As I expected, I never heard another word about it from Marc — "just another fishing expedition," I thought.

The ongoing government investigations seemed to drag on at a snail's pace and I wondered if Scientology's OSA operatives had infiltrated the agencies to thwart the process. Weeks turned into months and still no decisions were indeed wearing.

I thought the 19 page cover letter with numerous attached evidence documents that I submitted to the Quebec College of Physicians, was straight forward. It was a no-brainer for the College to declare Narconon's medical manager, Dr. Pierre Labonte, guilty as claimed. The formal complaint was filed back in October 2010 and months later, still no reply from the College.

Ban the Doctor — a Milestone

The complaint was directed to the 'College Investigation Branch' alleging 'Malpractice and Breach of Code of Ethics', urging the College to carefully examine all of the statements from myself, other patients, and ex-staff members.

I claimed that, under the guidance of Dr. Labonte, Narconon staff administered unsafe and dangerous substances and practices to vulnerable and exploited patients at Narconon Trois-Rivières.

In my lengthy submission, I referenced several College ACTS of 'GENERAL DUTIES OF A PHYSICIAN', stating that "Dr. Pierre Labonte, the consulting physician for Narconon Trois-Rivières, knew or should have known the health risks and dangers to patients who are admitted to this facility. He knew or should have known that no staff at this Narconon treatment facility has any qualifications or government certified medical experience." I informed the College that "Dr. Pierre Labonte is a Scientologist and subscribes to the Scientology doctrines, policies, and principles as defined in this church doctrine." I insisted, "This Narconon Trois-Rivières rehabilitation center is a dangerous health risk to patients who are under the care of Dr. Pierre Labonte and the unqualified staff, and as such, must be investigated for Malpractice, Code of Ethics Violations, and Narconon Practicing Medicine without a Licence." Then one morning in late July 2011, I opened my mail box and pulled out a registered letter notice from Canada Post. I had to catch a bus for work, but would go to the post office after my shift and pick up the letter.

Thinking back to that day is still an emotional moment I'll never forget … ever!

The notice didn't say who the letter was from and I had filed so many formal complaints, I had no idea what I was picking up. It could have been a 'Demand Letter' from Narconon's law firm insisting I shut up or be sued for all I knew.

I was tired after a long day at work when I walked into the post office at the back of a mall pharmacy and signed for the legal sized, registered letter in a white envelope. As I walked out of the mall towards the bus stop to go home, I began to read the letter from the College of Physicians.

The first two paragraphs explained that the College had concluded their investigation of Dr. Labonte and "Solicited the opinion of an expert physician on drug dependence." As I read the next paragraph, tears rolled down my face — I was stunned by what I was reading. I didn't notice others around me waiting for the bus and I didn't care if they were watching me. It was a surreal moment.

The letter stated:

"As a result, we conclude that Dr. Labonte had been in breach of several of his ethical obligations by associating himself with a detoxification center administering treatment not scientifically recognized in current medical literature, by conducting an incomplete medical assessment, and by keeping records of mediocre quality." And then I read the judgement:

"In keeping with the preventative approach that is part of the mandate to protect the public entrusted to us, it was agreed by way of written accord with the College, that Dr. Labonte put an end to all his relations with Narconon." Riding home to my apartment, I stared out the bus window, wiping tears and thinking about what the far reaching ramifications of the College decision meant. With Quebec doctors now on notice that Narconon is a no-no, "What will they do — how can they stay open," I thought.

The College decision was *the* turning point in the rapid decline and final demise of Narconon Trois-Rivières. The College had done the leg work by hiring experts to investigate and now the Health Ministry and

Human Rights Commission could ride the wave of evidence. I had met with staff at the Quebec Human Rights Commission in Montreal a couple times and it was very difficult to explain Scientology and Narconon to the interviewers. They knew very little about the cult practices and abuses. It was so tense at times that we had to take breaks before continuing on. I took them on a journey of baby-steps, giving a little information at a time, so they wouldn't be overwhelmed.

At first, I received negative correspondence from the Commission, informing me there were no grounds to proceed against Narconon under the Quebec Charter. Months of frustrating research had me up long hours trying to find a solution to having my complaint accepted.

Finally one evening I came across a decision by the Quebec Commission in favour of the plaintiffs that I thought was a mirror image of the abusive practices at Narconon. The Human Rights Commission had brought and won a claim against Mr. Coutu and companies under his control for the exploitation and violation of the rights of residents in an elderly care center.

The claim read:

> *Exploitation of disabled persons in care facility — nature and purpose of human rights legislation — care facility policy discriminatory for economic reasons — compensation for wilful exploitation and injury to dignity and self-respect.*

The important part of the Commission decision referred to:

> *The Charter forbids all forms of exploitation aimed at the aged and the handicapped. The Tribunal finds that the legislation does not only address*

> *economic exploitation, but also concerns physical, psychological, and social or moral exploitation.*

The wheels in my mind began to spin as I continued to read. My eyes widened because it was like reading circumstances and abuses exactly as it was at Narconon. *"Thank you, God",* I whispered to myself!

The elderly clients were forced to work without pay, staff members lacked the qualifications, and residents were regularly treated as if they were children and often placed into humiliating situations, and on and on. It was incredible how the situations were so similar to Narconon.

The defendant presented evidence that the residents 'consented' to how they were treated, but the Commission responded with "There can be no consent or agreement with respect to exploitation." Now I had the chore of presenting my case to the Commission that addicts in a drug rehab treatment center were defined as 'disabled' persons, just like the persons in the elderly care center were defined.

Then I found an April 24, 2006 publication,[1] *Canadian Supreme Court Says Addiction is a Disability*, that stated:

> The Canadian Supreme Court ruled 4:3 in favour of two men denied disability benefits for addictive disorders, effectively establishing that addiction is a disability under Canadian law.
>
> The high court said that government tribunals handling appeals from citizens seeking disability benefits must follow provincial human-rights codes, which define addiction as a disability.

On February 2, 2012, I filed a formal complaint to the Quebec Human Rights Commission for 'EXPLOITATION of a HANDICAP' and added 'Slave Labour & Discriminations' to cover all bases. The complaint named Narconon Trois-Rivières, Scientology, ABLE, Narconon International, David Miscavige, and "each and every Executive Director of the aforesaid entities." Narconon's law firm responded that students at Narconon were not classed or defined as 'disabled persons', but their claim was quickly dismissed by the Commission.

---

[1] http://www.northernlife.ca/news/policeandCourt/2006/04-23-06-addiction.aspx

Legal Battles and Educating the Community

Following two days of giving testimony at the Human Rights Commission in Montreal, I received a factual report in November 2012. There were five cases before the Commission from three plaintiffs, including one for 'reprisals' against me following my filing of the complaint for exploitation under investigation.

Commission investigator files were then transferred to Commission lawyers for advice. Once the lawyer's report was completed, a recommendation was presented as a "Resolution Decision", making a summary judgement and their decision redirected to the defendants. If the Resolution Decision was rejected, a trial date would immediately be set in Quebec Provincial Court.

I also filed a few complaints against Narconon with the Quebec Ministry of Health on behalf of individuals who were students. One was from a student who allegedly was being held against their will and the Ministry quickly investigated the claim.

Trying to have Narconon Trois-Rivières shut down before someone died was another task that drained me at times, but I persisted until they listened. I think accepting interviews with newspapers and CBC TV helped immensely to expose the dangers and also notify investigating officials that the public was watching.

The Quebec government had mandated that all drug rehabs in Quebec must be certified by a Certification Committee, and this was my next target for submitting a 205 page document to the Committee.

Narconon continued on, business as usual, confident in their online publications that they would receive certification with flying colours. When I read some of their nonsense, I couldn't believe they were so ignorant of what was coming down. Narconon's Andre Ahern was seen in one online photo with a big grin on his face, holding a box of documents in front of the Health Ministry to whom he was delivering the box.

I just continued to update the Committee with the deaths at Narconon of Georgia and Narconon Arrowhead, and forwarded current information concerning the health risks to patients at Narconon.

Narconon Trois-Rivières Shut Down by Health Agency

On April 15, 2012, I received a couple of Facebook messages that Narconon Trois-Rivières was shutting down. At first I thought it was nonsense or maybe an attempt to set me up to publicize it and then look like a fool when it proved to be false. I screen captured the posts, but waited for more confirmation. When I received another two messages that said employee lay-off notices were being prepared and students were being relocated, I posted threads on the *Why We Protest* forum, and waited. I really couldn't believe it was true, nor could the forum readers.

Then I received another Facebook message that the Narconon closing was just a rumour. When I read the post I felt so sick and weak and felt like throwing up. Even though I knew my sources were solid, because their past information had always been reliable, I began to second guess my forum thread. Eventually, the closure was confirmed and I was once again elated and confident Narconon was shuttered. What a roller coaster trip that evening was!

The last message I received from a Narconon insider said, "David Love has finally won." Even though this was cause for celebration, I did not see this as a game victory. I guess to Narconon executives it was a 'game', but to me this was no game of any sorts, victims were being abused and dying and in my opinion *all* Narconons should be shut down before anyone else died.

It was a tense time until April 16, 2012, when a newspaper published the news that Narconon Trois-Rivières was being shut down and all the residents had to be moved out. The media stated: "The detoxification center intends to challenge the Ministry of Health, but cannot continue its activities until a decision is rendered."

TV, Radio, and Newspapers were in a frenzy to cover the news, with headlines like *The Narconon Drug Prevention and Rehabilitation Centre in Trois-Rivières is shut down for 'dangerous' practices.*

On April 17th, the Quebec Health Agency released a statement at a press conference, stating:

> The Narconon detoxification center fails to satisfy 42 of the 55 criteria needed to obtain certification from the Quebec Department of Health, 26 of which are deemed high risk factors. This is the assessment pre-

Legal Battles and Educating the Community

sented this morning at a press conference by the Health and Social Services Agency for the Mauricie-Central Quebec region.

On April 18th, Paule Vermot Desroches, a reporter for Trois-Rivières daily newspaper Le Nouvelliste, interviewed some laid-off, Narconon employees.

> Sylvain Bérard, the Ethics Officer, said that Narconon had already been experiencing financial problems for some time, to such an extent that, in recent months, the organization had even been admitting clients with more serious problems of a psychiatric nature.
>
> Some of these cases weren't admissible to the program because it requires cutting off their medication. But the administration chose to keep them anyway. There were several instances of attempted suicide during the past few months. "By law, immediate medical assistance should have been provided, but management decided to keep these persons without calling for an ambulance," says the former employee.
>
> "We had no right to have a personal opinion. The only thing that mattered was their teaching of Scientology. Don't do to others what you wouldn't want them to do to you. This was one of their internal rules, but they themselves don't apply it. They have no respect for us or for the residents," says Sylvie Houde.

Needless to say, I was overwhelmed with the non-stop media interviews and forum postings. It was an incredible time.

Many of my friends and forum posters were calling me a hero and other kind words, but I didn't see myself as such. Countless people before me had established websites exposing Narconon. David Touretzky, a research professor in a computer science department, was on the scene long before I arrived, and his *Stop-Narconon* web page is indeed awesome. Another site, *Narconon Exposed*[2], was also an important resource. And of course *Reaching for the Tipping Point* (RFTTP), was a document heaven, exposing Narconon around the globe.

And for the catalyst that set in motion the eventual closure of Narconon Trois-Rivières, I give much credit to Émilie Dubreuil, the investigative reporter from CBC Radio Canada TV. In a courageous investigation, Émilie

---

[2]©Chris Owen 2002

"demonstrated the dangers of Narconon, its links with the Church of Scientology and its attempts to indoctrinate children with the principles of Scientology." The CBC video and comments uploaded to a YouTube site, stated:

"This report earned Émilie Dubreuil a nomination for the Grand Prix Judith Jasmin — the most prestigious honour of Quebec journalism. It is important to acknowledge the courage of journalists to investigate an organization that pursues and harasses critics." After travelling with me for a visit at the office of Senator Céline Hervieux-Payette in Ottawa, Émilie Dubreuil interviewed three Narconon victims from across Canada, and published the story in Le Journal de Montréal on March 3, 2012.

The closing of Narconon Trois-Rivières was a milestone, but many adventures still lay ahead. Some would be *over-the-top* exciting, while others would nearly stretch me to the breaking point.

Chapter 21

Pressing on into the United States and Ireland

The real voyage of discovery consists not in seeking new landscapes, but in having new eyes. —Marcel Proust

As I continued to hear and read about the deaths at Narconon of Georgia and Scientology's flag ship, Narconon Arrowhead in Oklahoma, I came in contact with an ex-Narconon student in the USA.

I met him online in December 2010. He immediately struck me as a very caring, yet strong-minded young man, endowed with the determination of a well-equipped army. He voiced a resolve for justice and a will to help others in distress. He is a man of empathy and compassion. He organized a protest at Arrowhead on June 23 and 24, 2012, and then promoted another protest that was held on August 25, 2012. This next one promised to be much bigger, with participants from far and wide. I confirmed I would be there with him for support.

Tony Ortega interviewed me for a New York, *Village Voice* story published on April 20, 2012 with the title *I Think I Have Scientology by the Balls* and now Tony was at it again with a story about the upcoming Arrowhead protest on August 25th. He was kind enough to promote the upcoming protest at Narconon Arrowhead to help attract a good turn-out.

I smiled when I read the last paragraph of the story: "Love, well — he's just going to be David Love." Events were happening so close together it was hard for me to keep track of what just went by and what was coming up.

One morning I received an invitation to an upcoming event in Dublin, Ireland. My ancestors are from Ireland and I was keen on seeing what the event was all about. Within a few short days, I was on the list of 'going' to the event, and was excited beyond words.

It was a conference called *Dublin Offlines: Speaking out against Scientology* — and I was honored to be among the fifteen or so invited guest speakers. The conference was scheduled for Saturday, June 30th 2012 at 10:00 am.

My flight arrived in Dublin on June 28, 2012, and was picked up at the airport by some activists, Pete Griffiths and John McGhee from Dublin, and others, who were there for the conference from California.

I arrived at my hotel to give Tory Christman a big 'Love-Hug' and settle in. Gerry Armstrong flew in from Vancouver, Canada, and it was wonderful to see him again and I enjoyed our time together in Dublin. Even L. Ron Hubbard's 'great-grand-son' was there and gave a very humorous speech — indeed a great speech!

The next day we all gathered for a protest in front of the Dublin Org, a pathetic run-down building. So much for Scientology's bragging of "Flourish and Prosper" claims.

The next day I boarded a train for Belfast, Northern Ireland to meet up with Anonymous member, Gina Smith, for a protest at Belfast's crumbling mission building. Scientology was quite offended by the signs and later posted their disgust on one of their 'attack websites' against me and other critics.

July 5th, I checked out of my Dublin room and flew back to Montreal to rest up for my next trip to the United States for the mega-protest in Oklahoma on August 25th. The number of confirmed participants was increasing daily and we were pretty excited.

In the interim, I was invited to attend an SP Party in Connecticut, hosted by Pooks on July 20–22, 2012. She was instrumental in my decision to get the hell out of Narconon Trois-Rivières. Pooks, now an ex-Scientologist and also an ex-Narconon director, was interviewed by the "CBC TV — Radio Canada. It was the 'Narconon Expose' video that I watched in my Graduate Officer's office — the one that inspired me to escape as soon as possible.

Pressing on into the United States and Ireland

Attending this SP Party was a lot of fun, with laughs, lifting of spirits, and the networking that was absolutely unexpected and incredible.

Also, before the Narconon Arrowhead protest event, Anna Schecter, the producer for *ROCK CENTER* contacted me about the deaths inside Narconon. After we chatted for a time, she asked me if I would travel to New York for an *on-camera* interview, and I agreed. Then she said, "Ok great, I'll email you a plane ticket and have you picked up at the airport when you arrive."

I was kind of stunned that she wanted me in New York on such short notice, but I agreed and quickly made arrangements to be ready to go. Anna sent me an invitation letter by email stating:

> Dear Mr. Love,
>
> Thank you for making the trip to New York for an NBC News interview with you. The interview will take place tomorrow morning, July 31, and we look forward to meeting with you in person.

My ticket arrived by email shortly afterward, and I was ready to go. It all seemed very surreal and I just went with the flow, so to speak, and arrived in the 'Big Apple' about 9:30 pm — with a limo driver holding up a 'LOVE' sign to take me downtown to a fancy hotel suit.

Anna showed up while I was still in the hotel lobby to meet me and make sure I was comfortable and treated well. It was an amazing hotel room, with a sundeck overlooking New York that was bigger than my small apartment. The next morning a limo picked me up and took me over the strangest TV Studio I could ever have imagined. We entered a big freight elevator with a rickety wooden gate that the operator pulled down before pulling a leaver that took us up to a big open room, warehouse type setting.

We did one interview in the studio and one outside, walking along the sidewalk talking. When it was over, I asked the driver to drop me off in Times Square, and then pick me up outside of the church of Scientology nearby when it was time to go to the airport.

I arrived back home in my Montreal apartment before midnight and back to work on other projects. Then all hell broke loose! Scientology sent out volumes of emails to church members asking them to "blast NBC" and attempt to 'spike' the show. The email stated:

Dante's Eighth Circle

Narconon is about to get a big attack on NBC news tonight. Same old crap, we've survived it before and will again but your help is needed. This is of course a Scientology attack as well. We got instructions from up the line to have everyone call in and complain about this one sided biased show and say that they personally know people whose lives have been saved by NN.

So you are not going to lie because you do know people who did the Narconon program. But you are pissed that they would portray a program that helps people every day and staff who bust their ass working twelve to sixteen hours days to save people's lives in such a bad light.

Now comes your part, we need you to call the station and leave a message for the producer. Anna Schecter. It is getting harder and harder to reach her (email full, voice mail full) so that is why I need someone like you, tone 40 who won't back off by a couple of barriers. You call 212-███████, ask for Rock Center (that is her show), you want to talk to Anna Schecter, she won't be there, you want to talk to her secretary, you do not want to leave a comment in the general mail box, you want to talk to someone in her office or talk to her personally. Don't use Scientology lingo. Leave a message and let me know when done.

Signed: Sigal Adini — Narconon Drug Prevention and Rehab.

Anna and NBC were swamped with calls and the staff was stressed. Then the shocker came when NBC received a letter from my daughter two days before the Narconon show aired. I had promised my daughter that I wouldn't mention her name to media and reporters, and I kept my promise. But now her name would be splashed far and wide by her own doing. Of course I knew Scientology had something to do with this, and they didn't care about her name now being exposed.

It was a scathing letter of twisted truths and lies — a letter obviously coerced by Scientology. Each page was initialled, as is common with Scientology statements. My daughter called me 'David' in the letter and stated:

When I heard about Narconon Trois-Rivières, Quebec, being shut down in April 2012, that was a turning point for me. It was then I knew

I could no longer stand by idly as David attacks the very people who helped both of us, not to mention thousands of others.

I was stunned reading the three page letter that supposedly my daughter had written. I had countless emails, Facebook messages, and even had written letters from her recently, and this letter, especially calling me 'David' in some sentences and 'father' in others, looked like a sloppy imitation of her. From an email she forwarded to me, dated March 6, 2010, I knew Scientology's Office of Special Affairs (OSA) was on her case. It was an email from her old boyfriend who had relapsed and was acting on behalf of Yvette Shank, Canada's director of OSA in Toronto. In part, the email told my daughter:

> This lady who is in charge in Toronto has asked me to ask you to write something about your experience at Narconon, and if you would be willing any other info on his [David Love], past shady dealings. She wanted me to make it clear to you it is not to attack or hurt him, but to make him get on with his life and to let Narconon to continue to help others.

My daughter stated in her letter to NBC, that "in April 2012 that was a turning point for me." However, on May 13, 2012, I was still receiving loving messages from her on Facebook, stating: "Thanks Dad ... I hope all is well ... love you and miss you." It was very upsetting to read such utter rubbish in her letter to Anna at NBC, but I knew what the letter was about and *why* it was written only 48 hours before the NBC Narconon show aired.

Then on August 10, 2012, I received a message from Tony Ortega that someone, claiming to be my daughter, had contacted him, questioning some things that Tony had written about my story on April 20, 2012 in the Village voice. My daughter sent me a copy of her message, stating she had never 'soured' over Narconon, and that she had never told me to 'kick some ass' while I was still at Narconon after she blew (ran away), at 2 am in the morning.

I found the messages she sent to me and forwarded them to Tony to verify what she said. On April 23, 2009, she wrote to me: "I love you and kick some ass out there." I could go on and on, tearing my daughter's letter into the lying 'Dead Agent' pieces it is, but I'm her Dad and she's my daughter, and no matter what she says or does, I will always love her — always without fail. At the end of her letter, she said I would be angry at her, but I wasn't. But I was disgusted with Scientology and Narconon for manipulating and using her to attack and disconnect from me.

From receiving loving messages and emails, I was 'disconnected' from my daughter, being told not to contact her again, and even blocked as a Facebook friend. This is what the cult if Scientology does to families. It destroys them for the 'greater good of their group' … whatever it takes to 'keep Scientology working' and squash negative PR at whatever cost.

Being 'disconnected' from my daughter, is such a sad thing for me to deal with, but I try not to think about it often. But, I do pray, that one day she will reconsider what Scientology's Narconon really is, and reconnect. Perhaps it will take a few court cases in the media, finding Narconon guilty of crimes and deaths that will be the change? I don't know, but hope is always something I believe in and cherish. I love her and miss our fun times and laughs, and would love to meet my new grandsons that I didn't know the names of for several months after their births.

I still love my daughter very much and I hope she gets some professional therapy someday, to deal with the cult indoctrination she went through at Narconon. I don't think she understands or knows the effect it had on her and still doesn't to this day — especially the mind control and brainwashing.

Although I refuse to attack in whole, what my daughter wrote to Anna at NBC, it did take me a few hours to provide Anna with documented evidence, rebutting the letter in its' entirety. I had to do the same thing for Joe Childs at the Tampa Bay Times in Florida and again for Nicholas Köhler at McLean's magazine for all their articles before publishing.

More than anything, I was pissed off that I was distracted and derailed from what I was doing for several hours over two or three days in total. It was a constant busy time of non-stop phone calls and tapping away on my laptop. I could not let this pull me down or hold me back — I just pressed on every waking hour.

The Narconon Arrowhead protest was only a few weeks away and I was in close contact with people in Oklahoma nearly every day.

I had already contacted the Oklahoma Department of Mental Health, Senator Tom Ivester, as well as filing a complaint with the FBI. The Mental

Health agency was responsible for Narconon Arrowhead staying open, and I sent them countless documents to review before meeting with them during the trip.

The online complaint I filed with the FBI concerned Narconon committing 'Telemarketing Fraud — False & Misleading Representations — Online Fraud and Conspiracy to Commit Fraud by Online Scams' over State lines. In my opinion, the cult fell under the jurisdiction of the FBI because of the 'Interstate" federal aspect of the crimes. I received a reply with a case number and password. While in Oklahoma, three of us visited the FBI office and met with an FBI Agent for a brief discussion about Narconon crimes.

Then we delivered a few hundred pages of documents to Senator Tom Invester's office and then off to a lengthy meeting with a group of staff at the Oklahoma Mental Health Department.

As soon as we arrived at my hotel in Oklahoma, a news crew showed up and interviewed two of us for a newscast airing that night. The hotel was very accommodating — by allowing the set-up of lights and cameras over at one end of the lobby.

Then we rushed off for another news show in a TV studio and then retired for the night — a busy day ahead for the protest.

The next day, three of us were blessed to be invited to stay in the home of the mother of a Narconon victim. They had lost their son, who had died inside Narconon Arrowhead. Her story tore my heart to tears — a terrible loss for such a kind, loving mother to experience.

The Narconon Arrowhead protest was one that many of us, including Scientology's Narconon, will never forget. Half a dozen or so gun carrying 'Park Rangers' were at their hut just up the road from Narconon where we all gathered before our march down the road. Apparently, a Scientology lawyer tried to thwart the protest, citing a few ambiguous civil acts that were discarded by the Rangers as nonsense.

Seeing 'Park Rangers' with holstered guns was strange to me, but in Oklahoma, unlike Canada, the Rangers have a wide range of policing powers ... above what I was used to seeing. It was an extreme hot day and the kind Rangers provided us with cold bottled water and assurances that they would instil a peaceful protest on both sides for all concerned.

More TV media showed up to film the event, but most notable was Mark

Dante's Eighth Circle

Bunker from Xenu TV, a well-known chap in Scientology circles. Mark has filmed dozens of ex-Scientologists and others for a documentary movie he's producing called *Knowledge Report: Scientology's Spies, Lies and the Eternity Prize*.

We met Mark in the Ranger Station parking lot. He had a face-wide smile — a really nice guy who seemed to love what he was doing. His camera was rolling and he filmed us meeting and shaking hands with the Rangers.

The parking lot quickly filled up within an hour and we were all lined up ready for our march down to Narconon Arrowhead. I was honoured to carry a special American flag in the march. It was an emotional time seeing all the caring people, some of whom had driven many hours to attend. Bright signs with photos of the victims were held high. A blow-horn was amplifying the song 'Amazing Grace' and mothers had tears rolling down their cheeks.

It was so hot that at one point, Mark Bunker had to be taken to the Ranger hut to cool down. The Rangers provided him with fans and some cool water to drink. He recovered after a short time and returned to the protest with water in hand. The Rangers kept driving by to ask if anyone else needed water. They were great bunch of guys.

Because of the heat, we cut the length of the protest by one hour. The message was clear and LOUD that Narconon was a dangerous and deadly place that should be shut down before another died. We drove back to our host's home and Mark Bunker came along to film some interviews. It was a fun time watching the lights being set up and people having make-up dabbed on their faces. I laughed as I filmed the entire ordeal.

My brief interview with Mark was about how Scientology uses Narconon as a recruitment tool to fill their bank coffers. Not all Narconon graduates who joined staff, also joined Scientology. Only a small percentage did, at least that I was aware of at the time. However, many took the Field Staff Member's (FSM) course. Once completed, the graduates could then refer people to Narconon for a 10% percent commission that amounted to about $3,000 per referral. So, in essence, they were working for the Scientology cash cow, Narconon. Some were building elaborate websites in the office next to me when I was a registrar. When desperate addicts Googled 'drug rehab', FSM websites[4] filled the search page with results. There was no aftercare program for the *graduates*. They just went right into producing dollar signs for the cult!

Pressing on into the United States and Ireland

After the interviews with Mark Bunker, we rushed out to do a taped radio show.

Chapter 22

Insane Fair Game: Dead Agent Attacks

"Touch me" the man says again and again. "Touch me."

In what should go down as one of the most skin-crawling audio tapes in recent Scientology history, we hear a church operative repeatedly challenge protester David Love to provoke an incident so that Love can find himself in a world of legal hurt. —Tony Ortega

A loud knock at my apartment door startled me one day when I was tapping away on my keyboard — deep in thought, focussed on compiling evidence documents for a government agency. I detested being dragged away from my laptop — even to answer the door if I was zeroed in on something important.

"Now what does my landlord want or is it that crazy neighbour again," I wondered as I walked to open the door. I didn't bother to look into the 'peep hole' to see who it was, I swung open the door to see a middle aged, casually dressed guy in his 50's or so.

"Pizza," he said and gestured the tiny box held in one hand.

I was immediately suspicious — especially with not seeing the pizza inside a warmer bag, which was strange.

"I didn't order a pizza — whose name is on it, and what's the phone number on the bill," I said with a frown?

"There is no phone number or name on the bill," he said, as he stepped to the side of me and tried to look into my apartment.

Unless someone waits until a tenant enters, nobody can enter my apartment complex without being buzzed in, after saying who they are, using the intercom to the person in the apartment. How did he get in?

I responded angrily to the man, "I did NOT order a pizza — goodbye," and shut the door hard.

I hurried over to my balcony overlooking the street and main door entrance with my video camera in hand. Within a minute or two, he walked out to his shiny car parked in front of the entrance, opened the passenger door and put the 'small-sized' pizza box on the car passenger seat. Then, with the car door still open, he rested his right arm on the open door and called someone on his cell phone with his left hand to his ear.

Everything about this entire event was out of place. There was no other pizza in the car, no pizza warmer, and no name or phone number on the box or bill. And this man did not look the part your usual deliver boy, nor was his car a cheap run-around heap. A clean cut, 50 year old man delivering pizza didn't fit, and I filmed the guy until he drove away after his phone call.

"Was I being paranoid," I thought after sitting back at my computer to upload the video file?

I hadn't lived in my apartment very long, so Scientology sending over a private investigator made sense. Scientology is a paranoid organization, and when someone they perceive is attacking them, it is normal practice to gather intelligence through their Office of Special Affairs (OSA).

"But, hey, I'm no big fish compared to others who spoke out or attacked the so-called church," I thought. I knew Narconon executives and Scientology in Montreal and Ontario were pissed at me, but I didn't think they would really start with what the Quebec SQ Intelligence police said to watch out for.

I posted some information on the forums and the video that I uploaded to YouTube, and the readers viewed it as quite suspicious.

After a day or so, I let it go and put it out of my mind for the time being.

But from that day forward, I took the advice from the police and Anonymous friends who told me to be careful and on guard from being followed. One forum poster said, "Buy a big dog, new curtains, and a locking gas cap." I thought he was serious at first and didn't sleep well that night, but was told the next day that is was a forum joke related to some other post.

A few days later, I received a phone call from a media person in Florida that I spoke to a few times, and he told me to buy a new, solid dead bolt for my front door, and be careful about unopened containers in my fridge and cupboards.

"David, if Scientology feels threatened enough or gets mad enough, they do crazy things," the caller said. Others were more concerned for me than I was for myself. "What could they possibly do to me," I thought, shrugging it off.

I was far too busy to be concerned about things that were only possibilities, and continued compiling facts and evidence documents.

A couple of weeks passed and all seemed normal to me until I noticed a mid-sized, white car wherever I was. The same car and driver appeared on my street, and near the bus stop I used. It was the same car that parked outside the ATM machine I was at in a mall parking lot.

One evening on my way home from work at a bus-loop, I observed a scruffy looking guy staring at me. He would walk behind me when I moved to each end trying to keep warm in the deep snow. It was blizzard conditions and I was filming the deep snow-drifts with my camera.

While filming the blizzard conditions, I turned the camera on my 'follower', and he quickly turned away, trying to avoid being captured in the scene. Later that night, I uploaded ALL the video footage of him to YouTube, and included the pizza guy as the 'star actor'.

I really didn't care much if I was being followed or not ... just wondered why and how long it would continue?

"Could all of this just be coincidence," I kept asking myself? "No, not with this paranoid cult — I'm not the paranoid one, they are." And just to be on the safe side, I took some more of my important evidence documents to where I worked and gave them to a trusted supervisor to store in a locked desk. It was a high security building with employee 'swipe cards' needed to enter the first door, then a 'fingerprint scanner' to get through the second door into the workplace area.

Scientology Dead Agenting at work — When I went to the August 2012 protest in Oklahoma, Scientology took out an ad in a local newspaper, paying about $1,600 to inform the public that David Love and two others were a threat to the 'Homeland Security of Oklahomans.'

The 'Dead Agent' headline[1] was:

PUBLIC INFORMATION ALERT —

Oklahomans for the Preservation of Homeland Security and American Values, (ohsav), international hate group 'anonymous' Builds Membership Base in Oklahoma.

… David Love, a Canadian citizen, (right). Anonymous member: internet alias "Intelligence" — (whyweprotest. net membership page #1464). He has recently been seen on Oklahoma television …

This alert is the first in a series of public service alerts brought to you by 'Oklahomans for the Preservation of Homeland Security' and American values (ohsav) and concerned employees and supporters of Narconon of Oklahoma, Inc.

Although I was stunned when I saw the huge, colour advertisement with our photos, I realized this was just a typical Scientology 'Dead Agent' attack and I expected more to come — even much worse.

Online Attacks Continue

While sitting in the Dublin airport waiting to fly back to Montreal, I was surfing for up to date cult news and came across the craziest shit I'd ever seen or read. Some crazy person had published the following attack against me.

David Edgar Love, Media and the Great Moon Hoax of 1835.

The entire story reads:

David Edgar Love is a product of our times, a product of our collective imagination and mass media manipulation.

David Edgar Love, as portrayed in the media does not and has never existed.

The Great Moon hoax of 1835 used similar methods of public "persuasion" to the "David Edgar Love" machine.

---

[1] Full newpaper article mirrored on smartpeopletoday.net

With computers and television installed today into nearly every home, the Internet can be used to create mass media "clout" — and "persuasion" of public opinion.

Cheap and easy access to public media has created and continues to support many myths and widely believed urban legends, such as the persona of "David Edgar Love" — drug addicted for 35 years, a self-styled and passionate lone crusader for his own sense of "Justice".

David Love is the "human face" of one of the biggest media hoax ever created, courtesy of the press, and the World Wide Web.

Historic battles for control of media such as television transmission, radio broadcasting and newspaper circulations have morphed into a worldwide megatrend towards ultimate control of the internet, and public opinion.

The media has portrayed David Edgar Love as having been subjected to abuse while in the care of Narconon Trois-Rivières. It is a smokescreen, a mask to hide and to distract people from attending to what is really going on.

Narconon Trois-Rivières is an icon for our times — fighting for the right, to continue to speak out against the powers that be, that lurk behind modern day pharmaceuticals, and pill pushing psychiatry.

Enemies of Drug-Free Life Style

In Quebec, there is the prestigious College of Medicine, together with the Douglas Mental Health University Institute and the Allan Memorial Institute, all still pressing ahead with psychiatric experiments that date back to the 1950's.

Contrary to popular belief, the Allan Memorial Institute is still operative today, pitting its strength and capacity against Narconon Trois-Rivières, by recruiting as a "mouthpiece" former Narconon student David Edgar Love.

It only takes a few deft strokes to create innuendo, half-truths and outright lies, that can adversely affect the character and reputation of those organizations (such as Narconon Trois-Rivières) who legitimately appear on internet to promote a more healthy, safe and effective way of living.

By means of propaganda it is easy to promote the least desirable specimens of humanity, the least attractive of human values as being role models for us all.

Abuse of Media

It is a daily war of bombardment and attrition. We are all becoming relatively disempowered in the face of transcontinental power games, about which we have little knowledge, over which we have no control.

We have become a world of unquestioning followers of the latest in Megatrends. With obesity, depression and endemic illness, caused by frustration of true desires — we have become a collective of people who can be very easily manipulated into supporting causes and issues about which we have no direct or independent information.

People love magic and illusions — son et luminere. People thrive on news of amazing events, enjoy reading the latest scandal. People love reading tales of deceit and deception, of cults and wicked deeds — it brightens up our lives.

Illusions, hoaxes and pranks succeed and entertain us because they provide us in the end with a sense of security and satisfaction.

The Great Moon Hoax of 1835

Life on the moon was said to have been discovered in the Great Moon hoax of 1835 — it was an exciting idea that gathered momentum due to mass media hype and involvement. When the hoax was laid to rest — people generally felt more secure — the natural order had been restored.

The importance of wide public media coverage in the context of perpetrating any hoax has in recent times become more understood.

The moon hoax was the first truly sensational demonstration of the power of the mass media that had come into existence after the introduction of steam powered printing presses. Before the 1830?s, such a hoax would not have been possible.

The moon hoax foreshadowed what would eventually become a central concern about the mass media — it's ability, because of its enormous reach, to shape and influence popular belief.

Later hoaxes, such as the 1938 "War of the Worlds" panic broadcast would bring even more dramatic and disturbing examples of this power.

Modern Example of Media Hoax

For a good example of a modern day "hoot", created solely by media power, see article The Great Marshall Islands Cocaine Hoax.

David Edgar Love: A Facade

David Edgar Love is a facade, a point of media focus — supported by a somewhat bizarre and purposeful "anonymous" underground movement that propagates and promotes civil discord and tension on an international basis. Like medusa, its heads rear up and subside — at moments appropriate to the global manipulation of collective opinion.

An underground "group" was formed in this way, created expressly for the purpose of sowing seeds of discontent among people with the practices of Narconon that is otherwise highly respected throughout the world, as a safe and effective alternative detoxification and rehabilitation services provider in the field of alcohol and drug addiction recovery.

David Edgar Love is a hoax, a pawn, controlled by vested interests in Quebec that create and promote illusory problems, so as to denigrate, and deride the drug free rehabilitation services provided by Narconon Trois-Rivières.

What Is Behind the Hoax?

Narconon is known worldwide as a reputable drug free rehab program. Established in 1966 and now operating in many countries around the world, Narconon is praised by many thousands of people, who remain drug free today.

Thus, the attention should not be on the smokescreen that is David Love, but on the individuals behind the scene who do not want an effective drug-free rehabilitation program to operate in the province of Quebec.

I had to read the story a few times and wondered who in their 'right mind' would, or could, write and publish such a ridiculous story?

"It must be for Scientologists to read," I thought, because I, and soon

Dante's Eighth Circle

many more forum readers, would be laughing our asses off at such craziness.

Then another story by the same author was published, but this time attacking me, Canada, Quebec College of Physicians, and of course, Anonymous.

The headline read:

> **David Edgar Love — Narconon Trois-Rivières Closed — Canada Caught Out!**
>
> David Edgar Love is proud today to have duped and misled Public Health authorities in the province of Quebec, Canada to bring about the closure of Narconon Trois-Rivières drug rehab program, in April 2012. Upon the closure, websites have sprung up, claiming David Edgar Love to be the "hero" of big pharma.
>
> The main arguments against Narconon in Trois-Rivières, Quebec, by David Edgar Love are that Narconon programs don't achieve a 70% success rate, and that the Narconon sauna protocol, as developed by L Ron Hubbard is dangerous and unsafe.
>
> The Hubbard method of drug free, human detoxification using low heat sauna, together with nutritional supplements has been successfully used to detoxify Chernobyl victims, rescue workers at 9/11, and police officers in Utah. It's scientific basis and efficacy is well established, and proven for many years.
>
> People might well applaud David Edgar Love, and his personal crusade to see Narconon Trois-Rivières wronged and brought down, with the acknowledged assistance of that international organization, of dubious repute, that has links with the enturbulant *4 chan* — the Anonymous Group.
>
> People might understandably be confused. Until they learn the facts.
>
> David Edgar Love is now completely discredited. Not the loyal Canadian patriot, born on the West Coast of British Columbia, as represented on his anonymously funded websites, but simply a maverick — a wolf in sheep's clothing — only too happy to take 'NarcononTR' down, for a fee — and to see Canada caught out.
>
> Where did Narconon students go, upon the closure of Narconon Trois-Rivières — to the safety of CCHSA accredited drug rehab facilities in

Insane Fair Game: Dead Agent Attacks

Canada as you might expect — that use quick detox methods of detox that are dangerous, and the Vermont method of drug detox that is known to be incomplete? Methods that fail to provide the comprehensive drug free support that is essential for complete drug recovery?

No, Canada was obliged to see the residents at Narconon TR, given freedom to make their choice, transferred of their own free will and preference — to Narconon drug rehab centers in the USA — Narconon centers in the USA that follow the traditional Narconon program as developed by William Benitez and L Ron Hubbard.

Canada has been duped into closing Narconon Trois-Rivières on the grounds that its methods endanger human safety — while in the USA today — its programs are widely lauded and supported. No one in America today is taking David Edgar Love and his claims too seriously — the Narconon program, as practiced by Narconon Trois-Rivières is widely accepted in the USA — and promoted throughout the world.

In late April 2012, Canada made a decision to effect the Narconon Trois-Rivières closure — at the same time as Narconon International was hosting the highly successful Narconon Executive conference in Tulsa, Oklahoma in the USA.

The program was well attended by Narconon centers from around the world — except for Narconon in Canada that was having to deal with "troubles" at home — namely its closure, as the result of the "furore" created by Anonymous member David Edgar Love.

The situation was not improved by the Quebec College of Physicians, having previously withdrawn medical supervision from Narconon students while on the Narconon program, due to the fabricated issues roused up by David Love.

Make no mistake, despite the vociferous "critics", (that would appear from David Edgar Love websites to be the vested interests that lurk behind big pharma"[sic]) mainstream people in America today support, recommend, and wholly embrace the Narconon drug free rehab program and support completely the comprehensive Narconon concept for complete drug addiction recovery, Narconon is at a grass roots level supported in the USA today in New York.

Many countries in the world today use and applaud the Narconon

> method for its effective drug prevention programs, and for complete addiction recovery.
>
> Countries that have fallen into the trap of discounting Narconon as a valid, safe and effective drug detox and rehab method, due to vested interests raising flawed "controversies" about it, have effectively denied this process to be available to their own citizens at a time when drug addiction poses a threat to human health, places a strain on government revenues and would appear to be an ever increasing problem.
>
> Countries, such as the USA, that have not been misled by the "controversy" that has been promoted by the mercenary "hacks" of Anonymous, get the benefit today of the most effective, and complete drug addiction program there is in the world.
>
> Canada and the Quebec College of Physicians have been duped; have acted reactively to the "hype" put out by David Love as the "mouthpiece" of those with a vested interest in seeing "drug free" addiction recovery programs taken down.
>
> If Canada is to regain the standing that it had, as a free thinking, advanced society, that is moving away from drug based addiction recovery, as is the USA — Narconon Trois-Rivières must be re-opened, and re-opened without delay.

WOW! Actually, I wished some of what was written in these two ludicrous stories was true. Supported financially by big pharma and government agencies would have been fantastic but my check never did arrive. Most of the work I did to help shut down Narconon Trois-Rivières was from inside my tiny bachelor apartment that I called my 'Cave' — a rundown, one room abode.

Following the posting of these crazy stories on an internet forum 'ESMB', Paul Schofield (Scooter) from Australia said, "Damn, Dave — you've made the big time! In cult-speak, you don't exist — that's all they can come up with. Keep proving them wrong, my friend — they're shit-scared of you now." Another poster was at a loss for words and just said, "Wow! Just Wow!" Over on the Anonymous WWP forum, 'Xenu Is Lord' wrote, "The funny thing is that this only would not sound crazy to a cult member. To everyone else it looks like a nut wrote it." And then I had a good laugh from a post by 'Auroa', "Aha!! I has been enlightened. Now I noes why the "Touch Me Fuck A Duck" guy wanted 'Sir Love' to touch him. He needed to find out if Sir Love was for real." 'Auroa' was talking about the nut-bar Scientologist trying to provoke me into touching him, or reacting physically to his attacks against me, in front on the Montreal church. I was holding a 'Tax the Sect' sign one afternoon when an elderly guy came out of the church and started talking, and eventually seemed quite insane.

Little did he know that I was recording the entire rant with a hidden recorder that I uploaded later that day to YouTube as soon as I arrived home?

Tony Ortega from the New York Village Voice listened to the video and contacted me. He published a story on June 1, 2012:

> **AUDIO: "Touch Me," Creepy Scientology Goon Repeatedly Tells Protester**
>
> "Touch me" the man says again and again. "Touch me."
>
> "In what should go down as one of the most skin-crawling audio tapes in recent Scientology history, we hear a church operative repeatedly challenge protester David Love to provoke an incident so that Love can find himself in a world of legal hurt."
>
> "He was about five foot eleven, balding, in his 50's," Love says. "His face went bright red."
>
> In a very Canadian exchange of charming accents and quaint epithets ("fuck a duck", the Scientologist says), the two square off. Repeatedly, you'll hear the man say "touch me" in the oddest way.
>
> No, he didn't want a hug. What the man was doing was a classic Scientology ploy, trying to get Love riled up enough to push or punch the man, which would then be used to arrest him and make him the target of a civil suit. (We've seen the strategy used time and again by Scientology's goons.)
>
> Although we don't see the man's face during the encounter, the recording of his voice is crystal clear and really quite remarkable. It may be the most interesting reaction to a protester since New York org president John Carmichael told a protester "I smell pussy" while a video recorder was rolling in 2008.

The Montreal Scientologist was 'stark raving mad' and kept saying over and over again: "Do me a favour, touch me — do me a favour, touch me you fucking bastard — do me a favour, I want you to touch me — do that, be a man — you're just a fucking bastard ... I wake up every morning just so bastards like you will touch me." And when I asked him his name, he replied:

"You go fuck a duck — you don't know what the hell you're talking about." Then he became even angrier and said, "You mother fucker!" I replied, "Your face is sure getting red, you're going to have a heart attack — why don't you settle down — you're stuck in an incident." With a bright red face, the guy just pressed on with, "Touch me — touch me." With the recorder running, I wasn't afraid or nervous, even when he did get in my face and push me a couple times with his chest. Even if he pushed me down, I was determined not to fight back, but just record and report the incident to police.

After uploading the video on YouTube, I had a copy made on a DVD disk and filed a report with the Montreal police and gave them a copy. The event was investigated and remains in a police file, but no charges were laid. For me, it wasn't a big deal really, but I wanted the police to see and hear how bat shit crazy Scientologists can be at times.

I came across a Scientology website one evening: *Scientology Myths 2.0.* And there I was under the Narconon page:

"Facts: Narconon Controversy — Agent Provocateur David Love" I had no idea what an 'Agent Provocateur' was, and looked it up on Google. That took me to a Wikipedia website:

> Traditionally, an agent provocateur (plural: agents provocateurs, French for "inciting agent(s)") is an agent employed by the police or other entity to act undercover to entice or provoke another person to commit an illegal act or falsely implicate them in partaking in the illegal act. More generally, the term may refer to an undercover person or group of persons that seek to discredit or harm another group (often, peaceful protest or demonstration) by provoking them to commit a wrong or rash action (thus, undermining the protest or demonstration as whole).
>
> An agent provocateur may be a police officer or a secret agent of police who encourages suspects to carry out a crime under conditions where evidence can be obtained; or who suggests the commission of a crime

to another, in hopes they will go along with the suggestion and be convicted of the crime.

The *Scientology Myths* website attacked and accused me of being "an anti-Narconon extremist who has been trying to generate anti-Narconon and anti-Scientology in the press," and stumbles along in untruths for church members to read.

The lengthy publication goes on to say I attempted to extort $255,000 in a demand letter and that I had entered their New York Scientology Church, and illegally filmed and recorded my visit. And of course, they published the letter my daughter had written to NBC Rock Center.

I viewed it as just another lame attempt to 'Dead Agent', harass and intimidate me, but to no avail. Before Narconon Trois-Rivières was shut down by the health agency, I was accused of lying and being bribed to give false information.

But all my statements were proven to be the truth, and the agency found Narconon to be even worse than the evidence I provided.

So, even though it has been difficult at times when reading the cult's 'Dead Agent' attacks, I usually brush it off quickly, ignore, and press on with even more vigor and tenacity.

In August 2012, I received some incredible forwarded emails between a friend in Europe and a Narconon staff member in the United Kingdom. These emails shed quite a bit of light on what Scientology was doing to 'Dead Agent' me and the propaganda Scientology was sending to Narconon staff members and their donors — the IAS.

Here are the email exchanges between Anonymous and Narconon UK:[6]

Anon:

> You stated that it was political pressure that closed the centre in Quebec. I see nothing at all there to do with the political pressure you mentioned but in fact it would seem the Health Authority closed the centre as it was dangerous for patients. Can you & would you comment on this?

Jim (not real name): (Narconon)

> Again, I am not able to give you details on what happened in Canada, but I can tell you that there was a criminal element to what was going

on. There were criminal motives and underhand tactics. I know that these attackers paid money to have people go to treatment with a view to spying on, and sabotaging Narconon.

I am not suggesting that what is reported on Wikipedia is inaccurate. I am saying that the conspiracy existed in the fact that the campaign to close the centre was long fought, and numerous in incidents, and that the incidents that resulted in its closure were very possibly orchestrated, if not set up.

There were very possibly financial incentives, or political incentives for the inspectors to go in with a preconceived agenda: to inspect the place with the intention of closing to the place down.

The fact that Wikipedia was updated so quickly (before the news had reached the media) indicated that those responsible for keeping the Narconon entry up to date had an inside knowledge on what was happening. It was not someone from within Narconon. It happened so quickly that it struck me as something of a jubilant rub of salt into the wound, from someone whose plan had come together nicely.

I know for sure that this is the case, because I have read reports and communications between the attackers themselves. They were delighted to cause the closure of Canada, and they are targeting Narconon Alberta, Arrowhead, Michigan and California next. I am 100% certain of this because I have seen proof.

The centre in Quebec was closed because of its political links to France. France takes a very strong Anti-Scientology stance. The attackers used a number of different tactics to get the centre closed down over a number of years. I cannot really comment on this because I do not know the full details. Trust me when I say that it was very criminal behaviour and criminally motivated, and that the tactics were underhand.

Big Pharma blamed for the conspiracy:

Jim: (Narconon)

In Quebec, there was either a new centre or there were plans to open a new centre to tackle drug and alcohol addiction. It is a centre paid for by companies within the pharmaceutical industry and one which

Insane Fair Game: Dead Agent Attacks

will, in turn, finance the industry by providing treatments which use maintenance prescribing and so forth. Obviously it is in the interest of pharmaceutical industries, and due to the vested interests described, of this new centre, that maintenance prescribing is used.

It means that every user going through these centres will begin a course of treatment which will involve their continued and perhaps permanent use of legal, prescribed alternatives to the street drugs to which they were already addicted.

To have a Narconon centre in the vicinity preaching an entirely different philosophy; not only actually taking people out of this system altogether, but also educating them about the dangers of it, so that they protect themselves and others in the future, is a terrible inconvenience to these organisations. It is a threat to their business, and also to their long-term survival.

I can give you a little more insight into the whole situation by illustrating to you the nature of the opposition. Scientology is a believer in the spirit being the most influential factor on a human being's health and wellbeing. They also have quite strong objections to a lot of mainstream medicine. This is because there is a tendency for doctors to treat a symptom, rather than to look for an underlying cause and treat that. So many of the drugs prescribed will handle symptoms that people complain of. Doctors are happy to prescribe in the mistaken belief that they are helping people get better. Pharmaceutical industries are happy for drugs to be prescribed as the industry is so incredibly lucrative.

Psychiatry attacked:

Jim: (Narconon)

> Scientology challenges this, offering alternatives to drug therapies which are very effective because they handle the cause, and not only does that negate the need for drugs to paper over the cracks on an immediate basis, but it also kills off the demand for drugs to handle recurring symptoms longer term. Of course, this is a huge threat to the pharmaceutical industry, in particular the psychiatric industry.
>
> This is one where the pharmaceutical industry is most guilty, as it is widely known and conceded that there are no physical characteristics

Dante's Eighth Circle

> to look for in the diagnosis of the vast majority of 'mental illnesses'.
>
> The Psychiatric industry is the biggest attacker of Scientology, and in turn Narconon.
>
> The motivation is money, because the pharmaceutical industry is one of the most lucrative in the world and Scientology has the power to turn the current think on its head.
>
> I will leave you to draw your own conclusions about why Narconon in Quebec was attacked, and actually why Narconon's all over the world are being attacked.
>
> We know that our attackers do offer financial incentives to people to get them to attack us when they might have a reason to — for example family members of people with grievances against Narconon.[6]

"Can you believe this crap — incredible," I thought!

So, not only was I an 'Agent Provocateur' according to Scientology's Myths website, but now I was a paid spy to infiltrate and sabotage Narconon Trois-Rivières drug rehab center for the benefit of pharmaceutical companies? And, according to these emails, I didn't do it alone. It was a fine-tuned, orchestrated conspiracy I was involved in — working in concert with others.

Citing "links to France", "criminal motives" and that I was paid to go into Narconon, was a nice touch of imagination to have Narconon shut down.

As one commenter said about Scientology and their craziness: "This shit is too off the wall and nuts to make up — this is how brainwashed these 'scilon culties' are!" I heard similar crazy rants from mind controlled culties all too often, and agreed that these manipulated cult members were too brain-dead to think on their own — or use Google to search for the truth.

Chapter 23

Spin-Doctoring Defamation Attacks

> *If attacked on some vulnerable point by anyone or anything or any organization, always find or manufacture enough threat against them to cause them to sue for peace.* —L. Ron Hubbard, Policy Letter of 15 August 1960.

I used to find it unbelievable how low the cult of Scientology will go to protect their image. It appears they have, and continue to, break all codes of ethical and moral standards — equal only to what the devil could think up or do.

Fair Game and Dead Agent websites are proliferating across the internet with outlandish attacks against me, insisting I'm a criminal, drug dealer, wife beater, smuggler, and snitch.

The author of one website, who, I think may have been drunk or high on drugs when they wrote entries in the *Word Press* articles, declares that I divorced my wife back in 1995. I was astonished reading all the blatant lies and misinformation.

In their delusional minds, they must believe I will become extremely angry and try to have the websites taken down or prevent someone from writing a book about me. In reality, I couldn't care less. What they have published is all lies and is easily seen for what it really is.

Example:

Dante's Eighth Circle

"David — he will attempt to make all kinds of threats in order to prevent us from publishing the book. He will most likely attempt to shut down this blog. That's what desperate people do when they are about to get caught or exposed." Attacks appeared on Facebook and the Anonymous WWP forum threads, but were quickly removed by administrators.

It appears that Scientology, and/or the private detective(s) they hire, work hard to try and dig up dirt on their critics. When they failed to find something that could damage my credibility, they manufactured stories as per Scientology policy, "… always find or manufacture enough threat against them … " For now, in this chapter, I will not address all their accusations, but rather let the publication stand as evidence, an avenue for redress with lawyers and the courts. All of their attacks against me have been saved, screen-captured, and downloaded.

When time and finances permit, I may entertain defamation lawsuits against the website owner, content author, and if possible, against Scientology's OSA and certain individuals involved in Canada and the USA. We'll see — time will tell.

Or, I may just continue pressing on, ignoring the attacks, and focus on helping vulnerable addicts and their families avoid being put in harm's way by the Cult of Narconon and their drug rehab scam. By far, this is my preferred agenda.

To bolster the appearance of 'due diligence' research, the Dead Agent attack websites have many PDF files of birth and death certificates of my parents, home foreclosure documents, and even a 1992 flyer document from a charity I directed. But, no documents of any criminal record by the author of the website are published, because they do not exist. I do not have a criminal record.

So, although the *Word Press* author posted documents trying to paint me as this or that, with a criminal record, they failed terribly to verify the facts. Just the usual 'Dead Agent' attacks to divert my attention in an attempt to intimidate me, which it didn't.

Most 'Dead Agent' websites are designed primarily for Scientologists to read, but they are also an attempt to discredit a critic with the media, public, and other Scientology critics. When I thought more about the attacks, the letter written to NBC Rock Center, attacking me, and other people involved, I began to put all the links together.

Spin-Doctoring Defamation Attacks

"There's millions of dollars involved, I don't know what to do," someone close to me said — this was one clue that still rings clear today.

These vicious attacks do not surprise me considering what this evil cult did to so many others. I consider myself lucky compared to what some endured. I kept thinking of what Scientology did to Paulette Cooper in 'Operation Freakout'. Scientology planned a covert operation, intending to have the US author and journalist imprisoned or committed to a mental institution.

The cult desperately attacked Paulette Cooper, in revenge for her publication of a highly-critical book, *The Scandal of Scientology*. Scientology ordered their OSA operatives to attack her in as many ways as possible so that she would go away. The cult wanted her out of their way and shut up forever.

"Ultimately, Operation Freakout[1] was never put into effect. On June 11, 1976, two Scientology agents — Michael Meisner and Gerald Bennett Wolfe — were caught in the act of committing attempted burglary at a courthouse in Washington, D.C. as part of the Guardian's Office's ongoing Operation Snow White."

On July 8, 1977, however, the FBI raided Scientology offices in Los Angeles and Washington, D.C., seizing over 48,000 documents. They revealed the extent to which the Church had committed "criminal campaigns of vilification, burglaries and thefts ... against private and public individuals and organizations," as the U.S. Government prosecutor put it. The documents were later released to the public, enabling Cooper and the world at large to learn about the details of Operation Freakout.

The Church of Scientology filed at least 19 lawsuits against Cooper throughout the 1970s and 1980s, which Cooper considered part of "a typical Scientology dirty-tricks campaign" and which Cooper's attorney Michael Flynn said was motivated by L. Ron Hubbard's declaration that the purpose of the lawsuits were to "harass and discourage." Cooper discontinued her legal actions against Scientology in 1985 after receiving an out-of-court settlement.

I met Paulette Cooper in 2012 and received a copy of *The Scandal of Scientology* book. Paulette is a humble person and a very sweet lady. We

---

[1] https://en.wikipedia.org/wiki/Operation_Freakout

talked briefly about the book I was writing and I cherished all her advice. I was blown away to have even met such a famous author, and the note she wrote to me in the book to me was very special and inspirational. Paulette encouraged me to push on and keep writing no matter what Scientology did or said to attack me.

Now, Mr. Tony Ortega has published a book about Paulette Cooper, titled: *The Unbreakable Miss Lovely.*[15]

> *The story of Paulette's terrifying ordeal is told in full for the first time … It reveals the shocking details of the darkest chapter in Scientology's checkered history, which ended with senior members in prison, and the organization's reputation permanently damaged.* —Tony Ortega

And I shall keep writing as long as my mind and body are able.

> *Never be afraid to raise your voice for honesty and truth and compassion against injustice and lying and greed. If people all over the world … would do this, it would change the earth.* —William Faulkner

Chapter 24

Roller Coaster 'Journey of Life' — What a Ride!

With peaks of joy and valleys of heartache, life is a roller coaster ride, the rise and fall of which defines our journey. It is both scary and exciting at the same time. — Sebastian Cole

I think if tears were a stairway to 'Heaven', I would surely be there already. Whenever I drift off back to being inside the cult and the events I endured, I still do, at times, have to pull myself back out of that very dark and evil place.

Thinking back to when I was a young lad, living on the waterfront, brings back serene memories. Our home was only a hundred or so feet away from the ocean and I loved it. I had a ten foot sailboat anchored a short distance offshore and went sailing on weekends and after school. Freedom for me was sailing over to a tiny island about two miles away where there were no people ... No fear. I could forget the dreams of Dad dying when I was only nine — confusion and sadness was replaced with a whispering sense of peace.

It was my safe island ... a place of wonder and adventure. I walked the pebble beaches with birds overhead, bears playing in the waves, and eagles flying over the tree tops. These were the beautiful memories that gave me hope of what could be.

Many decades have come and gone, but I have few regrets with my past, only that I wish I had known when I was young, what I know today. I tried to allow the sad memories to blow away in the ocean wind, but they remained. The painful thoughts I would try to bury in the sand and cover up, but they simply returned every time the 'memory-tide' came in, and the sadness of my Dad dying, clawed away at me.

Before moving to the beach house with my stepfather and Mom, I lived in a busy home, with Dad working hard at his laundry business and Mom doing the alterations on clothes. When I was really young, my Dad would bring me to work on Saturdays and have me brush out the lint in the pant cuffs. He told me some of the cuffs had coins in them, but I knew he was putting them there for me to find.

Dad had a fleet of delivery trucks and every afternoon when he came home, he would honk the van horn at the top of the hill. I would run out the front door and jump on his knee to steer the van down the hill into the back yard.

My fondest memories were holding his hand as we walked along to our favourite fishing spot only two blocks from home. These memories are ever present and I will cherish them forever.

Dad was very tall. He was six feet and four inches in height, but thin from his diabetes that required daily insulin injections. Mom said he applied to be a Vancouver Police officer and even though he ate baskets of bananas, hoping to gain weight, he was rejected as too light-weight. It seems strange thinking about it now because he probably would be accepted with today's policies that forbid discrimination.

He was born in Vancouver, Canada, and his father, 'David Love', was born in Ireland. I used to believe my Dad was also born in Ireland, but seeing the death certificate recently, shows he was not, only his Mom and Dad.

The story I tell now is the most difficult to go back to. It was a traumatic life-changer to this very day. I shed many tears while writing about these events and normally try not to think about them very often.

An Event that Would Change My Life

One dark evening on Saturday, December 2, 1961, my Mom was extremely distressed and called an ambulance for Dad. They rushed him to the hospital. He was only thirty-nine, and to me, seemed as healthy as a rock, but I was only nine and to a young boy, Dad seems like superman.

A few minutes after the ambulance left, Mom and I drove to the hospital to visit. I could see and hear Mom being very upset. She was talking to the nurse and doctor, and crying. I stood out in the hall near my Dad's hospital room and waited for Mom to finish talking. It was like time stood still and it took forever until she walked over to me.

"David, I'm going in to see your Dad, you must wait out here in the hall," she said.

"Mom, I want to go see Dad and hold his hand — please Mom — please let me," I said crying.

"No, David, you're too upset and your dad is very sick and needs to rest," Mom replied in a calm voice. I remember the event like it was yesterday. I could see my Mom standing beside my Dad's bed talking softly, but I couldn't hear any response from Dad. I was so upset — very confused.

After a short time passed, we drove back home and waited for the doctor to call about any news. I was standing in the living room near the front door when we heard the knock. Mom hurried over and opened the door and we saw the doctor standing under the dim light.

"No, no, no," my Mom yelled as the doctor explained my Dad had died — he was gone. Mom could not stop crying, and crying — the ordeal was so terrifying to me. Then it hit me. My Dad was dead — he was never coming home again!

I began screaming at the ceiling: "Why, why God did you take my Dad from me ... WHY!" I was so angry at God ... at everyone ... at the whole world!

Before the doctor left, he gave Mom a bottle of red capsuled pills to help her sleep. When she wasn't looking, I grabbed the bottle and swallowed a handful. If Dad was in heaven, I wanted to see him ... I wanted to be with him and hold his hand. But Mom caught me and I was dragged into the bathroom with her fingers shoved down my throat until I puked up the red mess into the sink. Some of the sleeping stuff must have dissolved inside me because I don't remember much until I woke up the next morning feeling groggy.

Mom was on the phone a lot, making funeral arrangements and calling relatives in Vancouver. I was a terrible mess and then was told my room would be taken by relatives. I would be bunked in with my older sister who was seven years older than me.

The funeral was set for December 26th, and I thought I would finally be able to say goodbye to my Dad.

"No," Mom said, "David, you're too upset to go to the funeral and it will not be good for you to go." I was not allowed at my Dad's funeral service or at the burial of my own father that I loved so very much. It was like having my heart and soul cauterized with a branding iron as I think back. I was angry, crying, and felt so betrayed and lost. One afternoon I was sitting on my Dad's knee with us both laughing, and a few hours later he was gone out of my life forever. It just seemed so unfair and I was lost in grief.

There was insurance on our home mortgage, so that helped Mom a lot. But, she still needed to take a job as a nurse's aide at the hospital to make ends meet. Much of my time was spent alone in the house and it felt like I was raising myself. Sure, I got the odd spanking and mouth washed out with soap from Mom, but as a young lad, I don't recall much else. Mom was too busy it seemed.

My Mom met my soon to be stepfather who owned a nice home down at the beach. After the wedding, I was adopted and my last name changed from Love to Forslund. I didn't care about the name change then, but when I was older, I often thought about having my real Dad's name.

My step dad was a hard worker in the Powell River mill and retired after receiving his gold watch for twenty-five years service. I would help him around the yard with chores and we often went salmon fishing. He was a good man and we got along fairly well most times.

Forty-three Days in the Hospital

When I was about twelve, our septic tank plugged up and I was helping my step-dad shovel out the stinky muck and replace boards. It was a hot day and the smell was gagging thick. Next, I yelled out in pain, "Dad, ouch, I stepped on a nail and it went into my foot!"

"Get out and go see your Mom right away," he said. Mom cleaned the puncture with hydrogen peroxide. It stung like hell as it foamed and bubbled, and she wrapped it up with gauze.

Roller Coaster 'Journey of Life' — What a Ride!

A couple days later I was in severe pain with a temperature over 100 degrees and my bones ached terribly. Mom took me to hospital emergency and I was admitted to a ward room. My temperature increased along with the pain and I was screaming for help. The doctors didn't know what was wrong and I just kept getting worse. I kept drifting in and out of consciousness.

The wildest dreams came into my mind when I was in a delirious state. One livid dream was of my friend and his two brothers, hitting the windshield of a car I was stuck in. It was so weird, but I remember it so vividly because it was like being in a movie.

I was in so much pain and making so much noise that I was moved to a single room by myself. Mom wasn't working anymore and came to visit often. Too sick to eat, and having intravenous tubes stuck in my veins, my small arms were black and blue from the tubes having to be moved to new veins. It was a hell I would not wish on anyone.

Mom still brought me home cooked food every day, trying to spoon feed it into my mouth. But, I would just spit it out … too sick to eat. Once every few hours the nurse would give me pills and the pain would go away for a while. But I wasn't getting any better … days turned into weeks and still no diagnosis. I think my Mom thought I might die if a cure wasn't found soon.

Finally, they gave me an antibiotic medication that worked, and within a few days I was eating pineapple upside-down cake with whipped cream. It was so good to start feeling better again!

I spent forty-three days in the hospital and missed a lot of school, but caught up as best I could. My sister told me many years later that the illness that had infected my bones and body was similar to what some soldiers had in the trenches. The nail that punctured my foot was full of untreated sewage … and I just happened to catch the wrong bug, I guess.

A few months later, my friend and I were sliding down a sand shoot by the beach and I caught my arm on a boulder and broke it in two places. My arm was s-shaped and hurt like hell. Mom drove me into the hospital and I was put under general anesthetic for surgery. It only seemed like a few minutes and I was awake again with steel pins through a cast on my arm. It wasn't a big deal to me, unlike the other hospital event, and I was not in much pain after the surgery.

Death and illness seemed to plague our family, with my cousin dying after a car accident, my uncle dying, then my auntie. I was jealous of friends who had a normal life — at least what I saw and thought was normal. Most had their real Dad and lived in a happy family, I thought.

But I was determined that this devil of death would not take me, and I would someday find peace and a happy life no matter what. After what I had been through so far, I had toughened up physically and I coped by hiding my emotional pain.

Colour TV had not arrived in our town yet, but one evening I was watching the Beatles on the Ed Sullivan show on our black and white screen, and thought, "This is it — I love this rock and roll stuff!" A few months later, my hair was down to my shoulders. I tie-dyed some tee-shirts and pulled on a pair of bell bottom pants. Mom didn't mind that so much, but when she saw my black leather jacket, she was not smiling, to say the least. She hated it! We began to drift apart and it became difficult for me to live at home. My 'safe island' days were in the past and I built new mental safety walls to hide pain. It was the time in my life when I vowed never to let someone tell me what I could or couldn't do, unless I wanted them to.

I moved into town to my own pad at age 15. I thought it was pretty cool and I got a job logging for great pay. But with cheap rent and pockets full of money, things soon went out of control. My friends and I partied often and by age eighteen, I felt like twenty-five or thirty.

Most of my friends had long hippy hair, and we travelled around to rock concert events. One three day event at the Strawberry Mountain rock festival was a wet and muddy party that had us rocking to Seals and Croft, Country Joe & The Fish, Hossanna, and a few others. Then we were off to see Janis Joplin and The Grateful Dead for a two day concert at a Stadium in Calgary, Alberta. The Festival Express, multi-city, Canada tour were a few of Joplin's last performances.

On October 4, 1970, Joplin was found dead on the floor beside her bed of an overdose of heroin, possibly combined with the effects of alcohol. Being the rock and roll part girl she was, her will funded $1,500 to throw a wake party in the event of her demise. I was shocked at Joplin's sudden death, especially right after Jimmy Hendrix had just passed. These two music icons died senseless deaths from too much partying and drugs.

Time To Be My Own Boss

In my late twenties/early thirties, I worked in a cabinet shop until I learned the ropes, then, opened up my own, and had a small production line of two kitchen units a day. After a few short years, I gave it up and moved on.

Over the next few years I worked off and on falling dead cedar snags and bucking shake blocks. The money was good, but I was bored working for someone else with no sight of moving up into something bigger and better.

I decided to move over to the Sunshine Coast and bid on my own timber sales, hire my own helicopters to fly the wood out, and make some big money. And it did work for quite a while. I had a decent 4x4, bought a 3D Cat to clear some roads and set up a camp for a few cedar shake splitters. Then I took on a partner for a huge timber sale with giant, dead cedar snags.

We usually hired a Hughes 500D helicopter with five blades to fly the wood out. It ran on jet fuel and could easily lift up to 1,400 pounds with no problem. The 500D was not available one day when we needed to fly the cedar blocks off the mountain, so I hired a gas fired Hilliard with two blades. It was like the helicopter used on the Mash TV show with a huge bubble on the front.

We could see him coming up the mountain towards us for his first pick up turn. Then we heard a strange noise and a crashing sound through the trees until it hit the ground in front of us. I still have the photos of the tangled mess and the pilot walking around safe and sound after the crash.

It was interesting work, but we finished our contract to salvage the cedar, so I began to look for other work. Eventually, I moved to Kelowna with my girlfriend and we worked in an orchard. I ended up managing four orchards and a vineyard, working long 14-16 hour days, seven days a week. A few months later, we were married and our son, Jason, was born. We would take him into the orchard with us and lay him under a cherry tree as we worked. We bought two duplexes, a small kiosk store in a mall, a small coffee shop, and a six acre parcel of land out of town with a 4,000 square foot dream-home log cabin which was half built.

To others, we seemed happy and successful, but something always nagged at me. My wife was the best, it wasn't her fault for my distress. But I just couldn't stay put, working the same job over and over again. I was bored. So, we sold off our land and business assets and headed back to the

Dante's Eighth Circle

west coast where I expected to be able to work fewer hours and still take home a decent income. The journey took me back into the woods bucking shake blocks for a fly by night operator, but as it turned out, he was late with pay or didn't pay at all.

Not happy, we moved to a place called Esperanza, translated in Spanish meaning 'Hope'. It was a small place only accessible by boat or plane, and operated by a few missionaries. There were about six homes of varying sizes and a boat dock with gas and diesel for fisherman and tug boats. I ended up being the maintenance person, where I did welding and repairs on everything from boat motors to the village homes. I really enjoyed the peace and quiet and the people were very nice.

After a time, I was approached by the director to consider attending a bible school called Youth with a Mission (YWAM), hosted at University of the Nations in the Okanagan Valley in B.C. It sounded like a good idea and I only needed $2,500 to attend, so I sold my boat and off we went.

The Death of a Baby

A few months later we returned to Esperanza as staff members and I continued on with my maintenance job routine, as well as boat trips to Native villages to see if they needed help with anything.

Our daughter Maria Love was born while we were at Esperanza. She was a gift from our time at YWAM. Our son, Jason loved her and cuddled her often. Our family was complete and we enjoyed all our special times together.

There was another, very special couple at Esperanza. John [not real name] was the chef and cooked for the church groups that arrived for building projects. Anna [not real name] helped in the kitchen and was a precious host for the guests.

I loved this couple and we became very close friends. They had two sons and two daughters, the youngest being a newborn. One afternoon, one of our boats rushed their baby to the hospital in Tahsis. The baby had a fever and was in extreme distress. A few hours later, the baby had died of pneumonia.

We were all stunned and shocked, not believing such a thing could happen to a family that was so giving of themselves, so kind and loving.

After a brief grieving period, yet another shock arrived when the director of Esperanza told the couple they would have to leave and move back to Vancouver. The director did not give any explanation as to why he was sending the family home.

It seemed ridiculous and unfair, without any reasoning that made sense. The sad day soon arrived when they loaded up the barge with all their belongings and sailed off. The director's decision angered me and I approached him with questions about why he sent them home, and why wasn't Esperanza being used to help more people in need. I suggested it would be an excellent atmosphere as a recovery place for addicts or others in need, but I was ignored.

Directing a Drug Rehab Center

I decided to pack up and move into Tahsis, a small ocean front town, with a population of only eight hundred or so. From Tahsis to civilization, it was an hour and a half drive over a rough logging road, then another hour and a half drive into Campbell River. So I thought being so isolated, Tahsis would make a great place to have a recovery home for addicts.

I rented a six bedroom home and registered Compassion Outreach Mission with Revenue Canada as a charity entity. We formed a board of directors and used the Tahsis hospital doctor and counsellor for the clients. It was a small operation, with only up to three clients at a time. Church members would take clients out fishing and hiking up the mountain glacier for fun times, so they could see how beautiful life could be.

We eventually moved down to a waterfront, 4,000 square foot home, next to the hospital. It was on the shore right in front of the government boat dock, and had a beautiful, panoramic ocean view. I was clean and sober and life was good — except for finances. I didn't take a wage for administering Compassion Outreach Mission, but donations covered rent and food.

To help out, I got a job at the Tahsis lumber mill for a short while, and then took on a new logging salvage operation on a nearby island. We cut yellow and red cedar cants. The yellow went to the Japanese lumber market, and the red cedar went to local mills. The company I worked for was a helicopter outfit from the mainland. It was a solid, well financed operation.

We even had a logging skidder barged in that I used to drag logs up the banks onto the road for the buckers.

The Helicopter Ride

I owned a crew boat to run the workers back and forth to work every day, and was paid a contract price for that, as well as a fee for all the products produced. Everyone was making good money as we worked hard, long hours. Hundreds of dollars a day were filling our pockets. We would sink prawn traps on our way to work and on our way home pull up baskets full of delicious fresh prawns.

While we waited for the Hughes 500D to arrive one morning, I continued to drag logs up the steep banks of the logging setting and skid them over for the buckers to keep working. It was a powerful machine with one hundred feet of mainline cable and three sliding chokers. But with constant hydraulic oil leaks, it had seen its day.

As I jumped back up on the machine, after climbing the bank, I slipped and fell to the ground in agony, not able to move. My lowed back screamed in pain, like a knife twisting inside. I had pulled muscles in my back before, but this pain was much worse.

I called out to the buckers working down the road. The noise from the skidder engine and three chain-saws were so loud nobody heard me. As I lay on the ground, the high pitched hum-buzz of the Hughes helicopter could be heard coming up the valley. By the time the buckers came over to where I lay, the pilot had landed, wondering what was going on. Within minutes, I was carried over and fastened into the seat — and off we flew, down the mountain to Tahsis hospital.

It was a small hospital with an ever smaller parking lot. When my young daughter Maria heard the helicopter overhead of our beach home, she walked up to the hospital. The screaming loud Hughes landed a few yards from the front door — with hospital windows rattling, and staff running out yelling to the pilot that he was too close and noisy. It was chaos! As the blades came to a stop, I looked over and saw my daughter Maria crying... because seeing her dad all messed up was frightening to her.

When I was carried into the hospital the doctor knew right away that I had prolapsed, lower lumbar discs. The nurse gave me morphine and still no pain relief. After a few months on pain medication, I underwent surgery to trim off the bulging lumbar disk that was pressing on my sciatic nerve. It was a long recovery period with months of physiotherapy.

I filled my time by taking a real estate course from the University of British Columbia. It was an eleven month correspondence course that I passed with flying colours to begin my career as a licensed Realtor and Sub-Mortgage Broker in Campbell River. Except for a few aches and pains here and there, the surgery was successful, and my back was in good shape. I worked hard to obtain many property listings, and closed countless mortgages for clients. Life was financially good, and I enjoyed my career, except for having to work seven days a week.

One afternoon, I was taking down a large 4 × 8 foot plywood real estate sign after a property sold, and tried to load it on my car roof-racks. As I lifted it up to the car, down I went on the ground with the same knife-cutting pain I felt with the skidder accident. After a time, I was able to get up and drive to the hospital emergency. Another back surgery to trim off a lumbar disk had me laid up for another few months. Once again, I was put back on the pain numbing drugs.

I was frustrated, bored and in a deep self-pity "Why me?" mood for a while. Then, an idea popped into my head. Why not write a book while I'm lying around doing nothing … waiting to heal.

Since I didn't have a computer at the time, I went down to the store and leased one. I then wrote and self-published a couple of marketing books. The books were about how to earn money while working at home … an easy, step by step process. I had a few hundred books printed and turned a handsome profit to the tune of thousands each month.

Once I recovered from my second back surgery and returned to work, we decided to move to Courtenay, down the island from Campbell River. It was the next real estate boom-town, down the island from Campbell River.

After the surgery, I started thinking more about my birth father. My stepfather had passed away and I wanted my real name back, both for myself and for the kids, so we all changed our name from Forslund back to my birth name, Love. Then we made the big move from Campbell River to Courtenay.

Although I made a decent income as a Realtor using my adopted name, the 'Love' name actually worked even better in the real estate industry. It was an easy name for clients to remember and refer business to. Then the industry started on a downhill slide and small companies were merging in with others to survive. Many realtors were going bankrupt, some leaving for other jobs, and it didn't take long before the numbers of working realtors were cut in half. It was a tough time for all of us.

I decided to get out while still solvent and started working as an oyster shucker. When I was young in high school, I shucked oysters at night and on the weekends and did well, so why not. It was an easy job, and the pay was OK, as long as one was fast … as we were paid by the gallon. We shucked the slimy morsels into a round steel container and threw the empty oyster shells into a wheel barrow. When it was piled high, we would wheel it out and dump the heavy load over a bank.

Sometimes I think I must have had some kind of 'accident devil' hovering over me. One afternoon while the loaded truck was dumping a fresh load into our bins, the diesel exhaust poured into our work space and a thick, dark blue fog filled the air. I felt sick and stumbled outside and threw up the ground. Off I went to the hospital emergency. Blood tests showed carbon monoxide poisoning. I would be fine if I avoided any further exhaust breathing, the doctor told me. I was back at work the next day shucking away and we laughed at the incident, but in hindsight, it was a stupid event for the truck driver and the shuckers. I could taste the diesel for days after I returned.

It was another busy day at the shucking shed and the wheel barrows were heavy. We were a competitive crew and always tried to out-do each other with total gallons at the end of the day. It was dangerous work, if you were not careful with the razor sharp knife in your hand. Boxes of bandaids were kept close by for nicks and cuts.

We were pushing out high production that day, working fast and hard. As I lifted up the two heavy handles and backed out of the shed to dump the empty shells, I fell on the slippery floor. Pain shot down my thighs and legs. My lower back was twisted in the worst way this time!

After a few months of physiotherapy, Codeine, muscle relaxants and Dilaudid, I was still in too much pain to work. Even walking was horrific at times. More CT Scans showed my lumbar discs were pressing on my nerves and the prognosis was grave. The doctor who did my first two surgeries was a specialist and called me for an appointment.

"David, I think I have a solution for your next surgery, but I'm not qualified to do it this time. You will need to have it done in Victoria by a surgeon who specializes in cases like yours," he said.

"Let's do it, I can barely walk, so I'll try anything," I replied.

My doctor explained that the procedure was called a "Circumferential Lumbar Discectomy with Instrumentation" of my L-4, L-5, and S-1 lumbar discs. The operation involved cutting me open from the front and removing the damaged discs completely and filling in the space with bone. I would then be turned over and cut open to install titanium rods and screws to hold my spine in place until it fused together as one. And there were risks. There was a chance of being paralysed or impotent, if something went awry.

Still, I was fine with his explanation until I went home and watched a video of the procedure. It freaked me out big time! The thought of my abdominal area being cut wide open and a doctor with a long chisel hacking away at my discs made me feel sick. Then seeing the pieces of bone hammered into place with a mallet-hammer did me in. I didn't bother watching the second video where the back was cut open and the titanium rods and screws installed. By the time I was admitted to the hospital the day prior to surgery, I was so stressed I felt faint and dizzy. The nurse gave me some Ativan to calm me down for the night.

When the surgeon checked my chart before I was wheeled into the operating room, he noticed I was dizzy, faint, and given Ativan the night before. Being concerned, he stopped the gurney and said that he wanted my heart examined before he would proceed. So, no operation! I was sent home until my heart tests were done.

A month or so later with my heart tests OK, I had my surgery, and was up walking down the hospital halls the next day. I felt no pain and was very happy — even laughing. But, I was "out to lunch" — stoned on Fentanyl, an extremely potent opioid, approximately 50-100 times stronger than morphine.

After being discharged I was taken off the Fentanyl, and sent home on heavy doses of Dilaudid and Tylenol #3.

Months extended into years on a rollercoaster of hellish prescription medications. I just couldn't seem to be normal or drug free.

We eventually sold our home in Courtenay and moved to Prince George

Dante's Eighth Circle

in northern BC where my addiction continued. I was off morphine but onto something more potent and long-lasting — Methadone. It certainly did dull my back pain, especially in the high doses I was taking, but getting off would be a nightmare.

I worked driving a 'Super-B' tractor trailer hauling pulp chips 12 hours a day. The methadone made me tired, and to stay awake, I used other drugs. Finally I told my boss that I couldn't drive safely anymore, and laid me off so I could collect unemployment insurance.

Not long after, I would be on a jet to Narconon in Quebec — And here I sit tonight, thinking back over my 'roller coaster' of life. A life with many warm thoughts and smiles, but also when least expected, reminders of much pain and suffering.

I often think of my 'coaster ride' as one of still being alive after all my accidents, surgeries, and addiction. And also, more importantly, I survived the 'Devil's Roller Coaster' ride down into darkness … and I smiled and laughed often during my ride up and out into freedom.

And what a ride it was! I am so very grateful to many I love dearly … grateful for being alive and I feel very blessed.

A while back, my daughter Maria Love, posted something on her Facebook wall that I love and cherish: 1Corinthians 13:4-8 — "Love is patient, love is kind — Love does not delight in evil but rejoices with the truth. It always protects, always trusts, always hopes, and always perseveres."

Chapter 25

Man on Mission Possible

In Australia there are not limits on what you can believe but there are limits on how you can behave. It's called the law, and no one is above it.
—Senator Nick Xenophon

Thinking back over my life, and especially my time in the hands of Scientology, I am torn between many feelings and questions. Although I understand how this insidious cult, for a time, robbed me of freedom of thought, beliefs, and even love ... I have grown ... and learned.

I have learned to expect the unexpected, but at the same time, I cherish how God has given me strength, wisdom, courage, and most importantly, compassion to empathize with love. Unconditional love for other people who have suffered through trauma ... escaped Narconon alive, and survive now because they received professional help and therapy.

Many ex-Narconon victims cope well because they surrounded themselves with a new group of people from Alcoholics Anonymous (AA) and Narcotics Anonymous (NA). They 'work the program' and have made new, clean and sober friends. Being around good people who care helps to overwrite their past trauma with healthy, positive thoughts. Their path of recovery becomes a refreshing new life of freedom.

Without all the help and support from so many people, including members of the collective, Anonymous, I may not have survived to this day? Through all these much appreciated relationships, we have knitted unforgettable bonds of trust. This is a must for anyone when dealing with the evils of Scientology's vicious attacks against critics.

Dante's Eighth Circle

My only fear and dread, is the possibility that one day my child or grandchild, will unwarily be lured into a Scientology entity for a free IQ Test, or Personality Test, and even worse, a free Stress Test with an E-Meter.

I used to follow Australian Senator, Nick Xenophon... and submitted documents to the Australia parliament. But what impressed me most about Xenophon, was his speech that included a courageous statement:

> *In Australia there are not limits on what you can believe but there are limits on how you can behave. It's called the law, and no one is above it.*

Senator Xenophon went on to say:

> Do you want Australian tax exemptions to be supporting an organisation that coerces its followers into having abortions? Do you want to be supporting an organisation that defrauds, that blackmails, that falsely imprisons — because on the balance of evidence provided by victims of Scientology you probably are.

I am an advocate for human rights and freedoms for all, without discrimination, exploitation, or abuses. Indeed, all persons have a right to believe what they choose. The important issues for me are the doctrines and practices of individuals and groups that cross the line into mind control and brainwashing. The forced or coerced slave labour, degrading confinement, such as the RPF (Scientology prison camp), and the dogma of the 'greatest good for their own group' at all costs is suppressive and evil.

In my opinion, these are the crucial aspects of determining that YES, Scientology is a dangerous cult of human rights abuses and fraud. It blatantly, with intent and malice, violates civil and criminal laws without blinking... without regard for human dignity or democratic justice.

One French newspaper article by Émilie Dubreuil, titled 'Man on a Mission' published:

"David Love is dedicated to preventing others from becoming victims of this scam. I help those who leave, I write complaints — I meet with politicians." Yes, indeed I have spent the last several years of my life fighting most every waking moment of every day, and it's been tough on me being so far from away my children. We miss each other very much. But, as Edmund

Burke said in a famous quote: "The only thing necessary for the triumph of evil is for good men to do nothing." I look at myself, not as a hero, not as a 'man on a mission' — just as a simple man who cares about people, and knows that good will win over evil. The "Bridge" — as in Scientology's "Bridge to Total Freedom"... that is built on lies, will eventually be conquered with TRUTH.

Scientology is a cult that shuns their Sea Org women from having babies, and if they become pregnant, are forced or coerced into having abortions or even leave the organization. What other so-called religious organization forces this upon their members? I can think of none... none that I am aware of.

What religion coerces their members to sign GAG orders before leaving — forcing the victim into silence, never to speak out against them or divulge their secrets? And if the departing member does become a critic, Scientology uses their confessions to attack and smear.

What religion sanctions the killing off of what Scientology terms "below 2. 0" on Hubbard's infamous 'Tone Scale'?

Hubbard states:

> In any event, any person from 2. 0 down on the Tone Scale should not have, in any thinking society, any civil rights of any kind, because by abusing those rights he brings into being arduous and strenuous laws which are oppressive to those who need no such restraints. — L. Ron Hubbard, SCIENCE OF SURVIVAL, 1989 Ed., p. 145

Hubbard goes even further, stating:

> There are only two answers for the handling of people from 2. 0 down on the Tone Scale, neither one of which has anything to do with reasoning with them or listening to their justification of their acts. The first is to raise them on the Tone Scale by un-enturbulating some of their theta by any one of the three valid processes. The other is to dispose of them quietly and without sorrow. — L. Ron Hubbard, SCIENCE OF SURVIVAL, 1989 Ed., p. 145

"Dispose of them quietly and without remorse." This alone should caution and alert governments around the globe to who L. Ron Hubbard was and

Dante's Eighth Circle

who David Miscavige really is today.

In my opinion, L Ron Hubbard was an arrogant bastard, claiming and publishing that Scientology would someday be the lawmakers of the land ... in his own words, he said:

> Somebody someday will say 'this is illegal.' By then be sure the Orgs [Scientology organizations] say what is legal or not. — L. Ron Hubbard, Hubbard Communications Office Policy Letter, 4 January 1966

Hubbard promoted the use of the amphetamine, Benzedrine, stating that it "often helps a case run." A *case run* is a term used in auditing sessions and processes. I wasn't surprised he suggested such a thing until after I read his 1967 letter to his wife, stating:

"I'm drinking lots of rum and popping pinks and grays." — L. Ron Hubbard in a 1967 letter to his wife, written during the period when he was creating Scientology's secret "upper levels." L. Ron Hubbard died a pathetic recluse, similar to Howard Hughes, with long fingernails and hair ... being injected daily with the psych drug, Vistaril. He may have fooled many with his pseudo-science quackery that he wrote in Scientology volumes, but, he didn't fool the lab test results upon his shameful death ... dying with a drug in his system used to treat anxiety.

Scientology destroys families ... pressuring members for donations non-stop at times. Families once together as one, are forced through Hubbard's evil 'disconnection' policy to shun each other when one is deemed to be a 'suppressive person'. In the Sea Org, children seldom see their parents. Welcome to church folks, this is an organization of human rights abuses that have continued on far too long ... under the guise and protection of being a so-called Religion.

The Mother church attempts to separate and distance itself from their drug rehab network, Narconon, but evidence documents show that they are one. Hubbard states: "Narconon is the 'Bridge to the Bridge' and Narconon helps get people up Ron's bridge to freedom." In other documents, it's clear that Scientology's Office of Special Affairs (OSA) dirty tricks organization directs and hovers over the administration of Narconon.

Narconon Trois-Rivières alone, before being shut down by the Quebec Health agency, had gross revenues of about twenty million dollars while they were open. Hardly what one would call a 'non-profit' and a charity when one considers the high salaries paid to executives and fees paid uplines. And whenever bank accounts fatten, bring in executives from Narconon International and ABLE to siphon off even more?

I may sound cynical and somewhat disgusted ... because I am, but this cult of Narconon is just that, a 'dangerous cult' that leaves a trail of death — and victims that feel they have been mind-raped.

Scientology's Narconon is now facing investigations in multiple countries and cities from across North America and Europe. They now face allegations for multiple wrongful deaths, misrepresentation, fraud, credit card fraud, conspiracy, civil rico [organized racketeering], and much more.

Earlier in 2013, saw the Insurance Commissioner's Fraud Unit and police, armed with search warrants, raid Narconon of Georgia, taking away computers, hard drives, and renting a truck to haul away documents. Three million dollars in alleged fraudulent insurance billing was in the hands of investigators and the Gwinnett County District Attorney's Office. Narconon of Georgia is now shut down.

So, Scientology may continue to deny allegations and carry on status-quo in their public and media campaigns to bolster their image, but the record stands on its own. They may settle wrongful death cases on the court doorsteps only hours before trial, but sooner rather than later, their crimes and abusive nature will be in the public record.

Once case precedents are set, Scientology's 'Narconon Empire' may topple like dominos faster than ever imagined. Quite simply, there are too many media outlets unafraid to publish accounts spoken from the multitudes ... that are now leaving Scientology in droves. Media and cult escapees once feared Scientology's attacks and litigation threats, but not now.

Some claim that David Miscavige is to blame for all the carnage and crimes, but Miscavige wasn't the cult leader back in the days of 'Operation Snow White' and 'Operation Freakout'. L. Ron Hubbard was the designer of such crimes, not Miscavige. 'Operation Snow White' had Scientology send up to 5,000 covert agents into more than thirty countries, including infiltrations and thefts from 136 government agencies, foreign embassies and consulates.

Some like to proclaim if David Miscavige was dethroned and gone, Hubbard's 'tech' could be restored to helping people, and of course clearing the planet and making their own laws to govern society for the 'greater good' of their group.

In my opinion, yes, Miscavige is another sociopath dictator guilty of 'high crimes' that would serve society best by being locked up for his crimes. Scientologists can believe what they want, but it's Scientology's abuses upon society's victims that must be stopped.

Since my escape from Narconon, I have learned and experienced volumes about this abusive cult and it makes me feel sick every time I hear about another suicide, another Narconon death — another mother disconnected from her child.

What will I do next to help and contribute to the multitudes speaking out and protesting? I will join in whenever and wherever I see fit and necessary. And I will not stop until I see the death and abuse ended.

Although I have long term goals and visions about what I can do to help, most importantly, my love for my children is foremost in my thoughts. As I told my daughter Maria: "to love is to feel and give."

"The most beautiful things in this world cannot be seen or even heard, but must be felt with the heart." I look forward to the day I will return to be near my children … I miss them more than they could ever imagine.

I believe I CAN have a close family relationship with much love … and still believe and act upon what my heart's desire … my passion to keep moving forward exposing fraud and publishing truth. And most importantly, helping others less fortunate by showing them compassion and empathy … lending an ear to someone who wants to be heard.

Chapter 26
Human Rights Commission Verdict

Never give up until Victory.

Following more than three years of Quebec Human Rights Commission investigations, testimony, and reviewing countless evidence documents, I was exhausted. After filing the formal complaint on August 25, 2010, the Commission delivered a 'Resolution Decision on January 16, 2014.

This was indeed, a milestone that I worked on night and day ... every waking hour wherever I was. At home, on the bus, shopping for groceries, and at my day job ... I kept researching and writing.

Thousands of documents were submitted, and two days of testimony at the Quebec Human Rights Commission. Finally, Narconon Trois-Rivières was found to be guilty on every allegation. It was a damning verdict with severe ramifications with 'Factual Reports' of human rights abuse violations that Scientology wanted swept under the rug. Here was an entity, the Church of Scientology, who had their own so-called 'Citizens Commission on Human Rights' — and they violated human rights, the very same thing they claimed they protected.

Now they faced paying three victims for moral and punitive damages, and horrific abuses. These included discrimination, exploitation of a handicap, psychological violence, hazardous treatments to health, forced labour, forced confinement, coercion, disturbing and traumatic treatments.

And notably, the documentary and testimonial evidence establishing that the respondent contributed to the financial exploitation of the victims.

These cases were a first for the Quebec Human Rights Commission, and at the beginning they were not eager to proceed. They informed me that "exploitation of a handicap" only pertained to elderly people in a care home. The Commission won the "Coutu" case with $1.4 million for moral damages suffered by the residents and an additional sum of $141,330 for punitive damages, plus interest.

I mentioned the case to a Commission investigator but was told this case was not about alcoholics or addicts, and didn't fall under the mandate of the Commission.

It was a frustrating few weeks and months with emails back and forth, not seeming to get anywhere to convince the Commission. The 'Coutu' case precedent they won was the very same circumstances and facts as the Narconon case I presented to them.

I studied the lengthy case for weeks using the 'operative' word, 'handicap' as a foundation for research into Canadian and Provincial case law precedents. First, I had to define the words, impairment, disability, and handicap. Often used interchangeably, they have very different meanings that I had to sort out and fit into my case. I knew an addict or alcoholic would have impairment when using — and I knew someone with a disability could have restrictions to perform an activity in the manner or within the range considered normal for a human being.

A handicap person has a disadvantage for a given individual that limits or prevents the fulfillment of a role that is normal. Although all the word definitions seemed the same to me when I first read about them, they indeed, do differ. And with the battle raging between my submissions and Narconon's submissions to the Commission, it appeared they were both travelling down the same path. I was so frustrated... "There must be a way," I thought.

In my next submission, I insisted that Narconon patients had both a disability and were handicapped. It was obvious that when patients arrived at Narconon that they were both ... not able to think clearly or reason, and could not understand or comprehend what Narconon staff presented to them for signing.

Many were still high on drugs or drunk — unable to walk straight and with slurred speech. But staff still forced a pen into their hands and the patients scratched their signature on or about the blurry line. The patient was then escorted over to the Detox Withdrawal Unit.

Taking an objective view as best I could, I concluded that addicts and alcoholics under the influence were handicap at the very least, and had a disability that prohibited them from functioning normally until they went through the Detox phase, and completed the entire treatment program.

Of course, this wasn't science-based treatment — only cult indoctrination without any councillors or therapists to help treat patients at Narconon. No doctors and no nurses were at the center. So, in my opinion, the patient would not heal from their "disability or handicap" while at Narconon. Many of the patients had coexisting mental illness and alcohol, drug abuse.

Narconon's lawyer insisted to the Commission that patients were only in the 'handicap' stage until they were out of the Detox Withdrawal Unit, then the patient no longer was handicap. I disagreed and went Google-Hunting again for days on end until the wee hours of every morning.

Finally, I found an April 21, 2006, Canada Supreme Court Ruling that would turn the tide in my favour for the Human Rights Commission to consider.

The court ruled that legislation under provincial human rights codes must now be considered by all government tribunals when handling alcoholism and drug addiction that are clearly defined as disabilities. Bingo ... I had what I needed.

"The court ruled legislation under provincial human rights codes must now be considered by all government tribunals when handling appeal cases by Canadian citizens applying for benefits, specifically, disability benefits. The decision means vulnerable people can claim human rights considerations and be protected by provisions under the human rights code before every tribunal in the country," said Kurke. "These tribunals can't tell people any longer to go away insisting they don't have the authority to deal with human rights issues." The Quebec Human Rights Commission had no choice but to accept the ruling from the Supreme Court of Canada and begin moving forward with their team of investigators.

I then studied the "Coutu" case precedent in more detail and presented

Dante's Eighth Circle

factual evidence to the Commission that was exact or similar to the case precedent. In the "Coutu" case, victims were elderly with disabilities, and they were exploited into forced labour, staff members lacked qualifications, and placed patients into humiliating situations.

Even though some of the residents consented to such treatment, the Tribunal found, "There can be no consent or agreement with respect to exploitation." The "Coutu" and Narconon cases were so similar in nature I felt it was a 'slam-dunk' position without any doubt whatsoever. I just needed to provide the Commission with enough supporting evidence documents for them to have an air-tight case. I decided not to give the Commission ALL the documents I had, just enough for a victory ... approximately 3,700 pages. The rest of the documents I kept stored in a safe place in case I needed them for a court trial.

After examining all the documents and interviewing the plaintiffs and defendants, the Commission found Narconon Trois-Rivières guilty on all counts that we had alleged ... and even more.

> VERDICT — Commission RESOLUTION CP-654.28: 654th sitting held on Jan. 16, 2014
>
> CASE FILE: C0686_10: "David Edgar Love vs Narconon Trois-Rivières" was resolved during the 654th meeting of the Complaints Committee held on January 16, 2014, in accordance with section 61 of the Charter of human rights and freedoms (R.S.Q., c. C-12), and in accordance with the Regulation respecting the handling of complaints and the procedure applicable to the investigations of the Commission des droits de la personne.
>
> CONSIDERING that the Commission des droits de la personne et des droits de la jeunesse shall promote and uphold, by every appropriate measure, the principles contained in the Charter of human rights and freedoms;
>
> CONSIDERING that, among the responsibilities listed under section 71 of the Charter, the Commission shall, in particular, investigate on its own initiative or following receipt of a complaint, any situation which "appears to the Commission to be either a case of discrimination within the meaning of sections 10 to 19, ... õr a violation of the right of aged or handicapped persons against exploitation enunciated in the first

paragraph of section 48";

CONSIDERING that on August 25, 2010, the complainant, who suffers from drug addiction, filed a complaint before the Commission, alleging to be a victim of economic discrimination, humiliation, verbal and psychological violence by Narconon Trois-Rivières, a legal person that had been welcoming adults suffering from drug and alcohol addiction since 2001;

CONSIDERING, more specifically, that the complainant criticized the respondent for submitting him to treatments potentially hazardous to his health, and without adequate medical supervision by qualified professionals, for forcing him to perform various tasks without pay, for forcing him to undergo disturbing and traumatic treatments, and for forcing him to submit to indoctrination measures without his knowledge and against his will;

CONSIDERING the investigation conducted by the Commission in the present case;

CONSIDERING that upon completion of this investigation, the respondent, Narconon Trois-Rivières, has received a statement of the relevant facts and has been invited to produce its comments, in accordance with section 7 of the Regulation respecting the handling of complaints and the procedure applicable to the investigations;

CONSIDERING that the purpose of the Commission's investigation is to seek any evidence, in accordance with the first paragraph of section 78 of the Charter, allowing it to decide whether it is expedient to foster the negotiation of a settlement between the parties, to propose the submission of the dispute to arbitration or to refer any unsettled issue to a tribunal;

CONSIDERING, in accordance with section 79 of the Charter, that the Commission may also propose, taking into account the public interest and the interest of the victim, any measure of redress, such as the admission of the violation of a right, the cessation of the act complained of, the performance of any act or the payment of compensation or punitive damages, within such time as it fixes;

CONSIDERING under section 80 of the Charter, where the measure of redress proposed by the Commission has not been implemented within the allotted time, the Commission may apply to a tribunal "to obtain, where consistent with the public interest, any appropriate measure against the person at fault or to demand, in favour of the victim, any measure of redress it considers appropriate at that time";

CONSIDERING, in this case, that the Commission is of the opinion that the evidence before it at the end of the investigation regarding the allegation of exploitation toward Mr. David Edgar Love is sufficient to apply to a tribunal;

CONSIDERING, notably, the documentary and testimonial evidence establishing that the respondent contributed to the financial exploitation of the victim, who was in a vulnerable position, by

- Charging him considerable amounts for a detoxification program which was not scientifically approved and which involved health and safety hazards;
- Failing to provide him with care suited to his medical condition, despite the sums he paid;
- Providing information, before and during treatment, which could be misleading as to the likelihood of a successful outcome, and which gave the impression that the results were guaranteed;
- Charging him large sums for a service provided by unqualified people;
- Forcing him to work and perform various tasks without pay.

CONSIDERING that the evidence also established that the respondent contributed to the victim's exploitation in the form of abuse, notably by

- Forcing him to submit to humiliating and degrading practices;
- Failing to properly bear the responsibility for confidential information obtained from the complainant after prompting him to open up about personal aspects of his life;

Human Rights Commission Verdict

- Using controversial teaching methods that were not based on any scientific study;

- Submitting him to poor living and food conditions;

- Submitting him to forced confinement and coercion.

CONSIDERING that the Commission is also of the opinion that it is necessary to propose measures of redress based on section 79 of the Charter, prior to applying to a tribunal;

FOR THESE REASONS, taking into account the public interest and the interest of the victim, the Commission proposes the following measure of redress to the respondent, Narconon Trois-Rivières, namely to:

PAY the victim, David Edgar Love, a sum of $45,000 (forty-five thousand dollars) distributed as follows:

a) A sum of $25,000 (twenty-five thousand dollars) in moral damages on account of the violation of the victim's rights under section 4, 10 and 48 of the Charter;

b) A sum $20,000 (twenty thousand dollars) as punitive damages for the unlawful and intentional interference with the victim's rights.

The Commission des droits de la personne et des droits de la jeunesse is requesting that the respondent, Narconon Trois-Rivières:

MEET the aforementioned proposed measure of redress, on or before Friday, March 21, 2014 at 3 p.m.

Should the respondent fail to implement the above recommendation, within the specified time frame, the Commission MANDATES its Litigation Department to apply to a tribunal to obtain, where consistent with the public interest, any appropriate measure or to claim, in favour of the victim, any measure it considers appropriate.

Resolution passed unanimously by the members of the Complaints committee at its 654th sitting held on January 16, 2014 as Resolution CP-654.28.

Dante's Eighth Circle

I won on all counts claimed and so did the other two victims. My total was $45,000, one victim was the same at $45,000, and the third victim was awarded a total of $50,000. All three combined totalled a sum of $140,000.

I was very happy ... we had done what no other had ever succeeded in doing against a Scientology entity. We convinced a Human Rights Commission to find Narconon responsible for violating our human rights and freedoms. And for Narconon, the Resolution ordered them to pay the victims for moral and punitive damages.

When I received the Resolution Decision from the Commission, I stood up from my laptop and paced back and forth in my tiny apartment ... not really believing what I had just read.

I believe that I won because of what Robert Kennedy said about "standing up for an ideal ... improve the lot of others ... tiny ripples of hope ... sweeping down the mightiest of oppression and resistance." Yes, I believed it could be done and if it was right and just ... it would be done.

"It is from numberless diverse acts of courage and belief that human history is shaped. Each time a man stands up for an ideal, or acts to improve the lot of others, or strikes out against injustice, he sends forth a tiny ripple of hope, and crossing each other from a million different centers of energy and daring those ripples build a current which can sweep down the mightiest walls of oppression and resistance." — Robert F. Kennedy

However, the human right's commission decision was not binding on Narconon, and they fought tooth and nail to have the decision kept quiet, never to be seen by the public or media. Scientology appointed a Quebec law firm that appeared to be unfamiliar with who and what this cult does and how they operate. As usual, and in many cases like this, their lawyers representing Narconon Trois-Rivières were being dangled like puppets.

One of my Montreal lawyers from the Commission sent me an email, stating:

> Dear Mr. Love, as you can imagine, I still haven't heard from Narconon's attorneys yet. Three different scenarios are possible.
>
> 1. They will contact me this afternoon with a new proposition for settlement;
>
> 2. They will contact me this afternoon to request a new extension;

Human Rights Commission Verdict

> 3. They will remain silent. If they request an extension, would you agree to a 2-3 days delay? Would you agree to wait until Monday or Tuesday to hear their proposition? The only option that remains, otherwise, is to go to court with all the consequences attached to such a decision.

Narconon's lawyers had already insisted they would file for bankruptcy rather than face a court trial that, without a doubt, they would lose. They knew that exposing all their crimes and human rights abuses on the public record for the world to see and use as case precedents would have serious ramifications.

Following a two hour meeting with a couple of Human Rights Commission lawyers, I could tell they did not want to pursue any of the three cases further into a full-blown trial. In the same email, my lawyers said:

> But we have to be realistic. If Narconon agrees to pay some damages, it will be in exchange of your confidentiality (from the three of you). If we go to court, the case will then be public and the chances that they will agree to pay damages are almost void. We will see how the situation evolves this afternoon. Be certain that I will keep you up to date of any developments. — Stéphanie Fournier, avocate.

In my deepest being, I felt that Narconon's lawyers were being micromanaged by Scientology lawyers in California and/or Clearwater by their dirty tricks, Office of Special Affairs rat-nest. Scientology in-house lawyer, Kendrick Moxon, had a couple of brief email exchanges with me over the course this ordeal, and I suspect that David Miscavige, had his wee fingers in this giant mess. The proceedings and negotiations seemed like someone with clout, with a narcissistic behaviour disorder was directing the pending outcome in Montreal.

At the two hour meeting with my Commission appointed lawyers, I was informed that the lawyers representing Narconon told my lawyers that their client was so broke that they [the lawyers] feared they would not even be reimbursed for the cab fare to the meeting they had with my lawyers earlier that week.

I was vehemently opposed to any confidentiality, non-disclosure, or Gag-Order agreement that would prevent me from speaking about the human

Dante's Eighth Circle

rights violations and horrific abuses at Narconon.

Another email arrived from my lawyer, stating:

> Good day Mr. Love, here is a summary of the latest developments, as requested: Narconon's attorneys confirmed to us that Narconon do not want to negotiate "individually." They want three settlements or nothing. They confirmed that the confidentiality clause is at stake; The attorneys provided us with new information regarding the financial situation of Narconon. We learned that there is many judgments ordered against Narconon totalizing over half millions dollars (mostly for unpaid income taxes). They confirmed to us that if there is no settlement, Narconon is going to declare bankruptcy, which, as I explained to you previously, will limit our actions if we want to go to trial. In the case of a bankruptcy, the Commission will legally be under the obligation to stop all legal proceedings; As I am writing this email, I still haven't heard about Narconon's attorneys. We are still waiting to know what will be their answer to your counter offer. — Stéphanie Fournier, avocate.

My counter offer was quite simple and to the point. I said, "Sure, inform Narconon's lawyers that I will sign a "Limited" non-disclosure agreement, on my terms, not theirs." I expressed to my lawyer that I could not live with having my intrinsic human rights and freedoms violated once again by this insidious cult by signing away my freedom of speech. Being shackled in chains by a non-disclosure agreement was against every fibre in my mind. Sure, I could have walked away with twenty or thirty thousand dollars in my pocket ... or perhaps even more, but could I look at myself in the mirror each morning and feel at peace ... feel that I had done the right thing ... or more likely than not, feel like my soul had been bought by the devil?

It was taking Narconon's lawyers more time than normal to respond to my lawyer, especially considering I had the right to send the Commission's verdict to the media at any time. It became obvious they were stalling and acting in bad faith — something that I did expect every step of the way.

Even my lawyer, Stephanie Fournier, was becoming quite frustrated, as seen in the tell-tale email excerpt during negotiations, "As you can imagine, I still haven't heard from Narconon's attorneys yet." Scientology and their cult drug rehab, Narconon, were bluffing and I knew they were without question.

"Narconon declare bankruptcy," I asked myself? The Commission lawyers believed they could and would if I pressed too hard or didn't sign a Gag-Order. Right from the beginning of years of investigations, it was like pulling teeth for them to understand and believe that what I was saying was true. It took thousands of documents just for them to wrap 'part' of their minds around the big picture — "they wouldn't understand, no matter how hard I tried," I thought.

Of course, I had still not submitted all the documents I had — those I would save until the end, catching the cult witnesses in lies under oath on cross-examination if we ever arrived in a courtroom.

So, here I am in their waiting 'game' — a cult orchestrated tactic of "stall the three plaintiffs" and see if David Love caves into the pressure from the other two. But I wasn't being coerced in any way whatsoever by the other two plaintiffs to sign the Gag-Order. The other two were just as disgusted as I was with Narconon's pittance offer to settle and go away. I wanted Narconon Trois-Rivières in a Montreal courtroom — on trial for their advertised false "Success Rate" — their "Forced labour practices" — their "Forced confinement and coercion" as well as a raft-load of other misrepresentations, fraud, and abuse that should have led to criminal charges, in my opinion.

Having the Quebec Human Rights Commission haul Narconon Trois-Rivières into a courtroom would have been David Miscavige's worst nightmare. Why? Because Narconon International, ABLE Canada, and the Church of Scientology Montreal, all had members working at, or directing and administering the Narconon program in Trois-Rivières. I knew that these Scientology entities, and the individuals, could be 'Served' with a subpoena to appear as witnesses and be deposed.

Also, the 'Office of Special Affairs' director in Canada, Yvette Shank, who was not only at Narconon Trois-Rivières on occasion, but also involved with the operations, could be facing a sit-down in the courtroom. I was in a dead-lock with my Commission lawyer, insisting that I would not sign any confidentiality agreement. My lawyer continued to insist Narconon would declare bankruptcy if I didn't sign.

"It's all three sign or nobody will receive compensation," said my lawyer.

Dante's Eighth Circle

I kept asking myself the question, "Should I call Narconon's bluff, knowing that they would dread having their 'books' subject to being scrutinized by a 'Trustee in Bankruptcy' and the Courts if I filed a motion."

According to Quebec civil code, I knew that any interested person may file an objection to having the discharge [bankruptcy] take place. Anyone could have Narconon's 'discharge' stalled and request a forensic audit. Having Revenue Canada investigate the finances, banking, and books of Narconon Trois-Rivières, could open an ugly can of worms that I believed Scientology and Narconon would rather avoid.

Following days and weeks of waiting for Narconon to act in good faith, and offer a reasoned settlement with a limited non-disclosure, I called their bluff and said: "NO, I want you [my lawyer] to take my case to court — I am not signing what they want." I recorded the phone call and uploaded part of it to YouTube that same night.

The next morning I received an email from my lawyer, stating:

> Mr. Love, I was informed, earlier this morning that yesterday, unbeknownst to me, you recorded our privileged phone conversation and that you posted it in a video on YouTube/Facebook. This is a serious breach of confidence. Meanwhile, before being informed of your actions, I talked to Narconon's attorneys and convinced them to increase their propositions for settlement. Furthermore, I have convinced them to offer you the same amount of money than the one they propose to the two other victims. I want to know what your intentions are by the end of the day, by email.

I replied by email from my cell phone browser within two hours, stating:

> Dear Stephanie Fournier, Lawyer — The video I posted is not of our two way conversation. The video is only my voice instructing/directing you of my feelings and intentions NOT to accept or sign any non-disclosure agreement. You stated to me that Narconon's FINAL offer, as they instructed you, was their FINAL OFFER and insisted it was no deal unless I signed a non-nondisclosure agreement. I will not sign a non-disclosure agreement. Narconon executives still have the link to the HATE website against me right now! I have not breached our Lawyer/ Client confidentiality because it is ONLY my voice in the

Video. I informed [one other plaintiff] about my intention not to sign the non-disclosure agreement and [they] sent me a written message stating:

"Go for it, publish your book now ... there is no non-disclosure signed ... they snooze, they lose."

In your email today, you only mention an increase in compensation, but no mention if Narconon has rescinded their demand for a non-disclosure? I reiterate my position from yesterday, and respectfully request the Commission move forward with their Charter Mandate and proceed to Court. Thank you and I look forward to your reply. — David Love

I decided to hold my ground and call their bluff concerning Narconon threatening to file for bankruptcy and their demand that ALL three plaintiffs must sign a non-disclosure or no deal. Over the next few weeks of submissions back and forth with the Human Rights Commission, including my appeal to the President of the Commission and the Quebec Ministry of Justice office in Quebec City, I was informed the Commission would cease representing me.

The Commission lawyer was under investigation and had to recuse herself from all three cases, and was replaced with another to proceed with the other two victim's cases. Narconon's threats to file for bankruptcy were just hot air — a bluff, and their demand that all three or none was a bluff. The new Commission lawyer negotiated a settlement with the other two plaintiffs who received approximately 50% of the awarded $100,000 for moral and punitive damages — split between the two.

Now I was in a position to do what I insisted the Commission do in the first place — not only hold Narconon Trois-Rivières responsible, but also the Church of Scientology Montreal, and the executives for negligence.

According to Quebec civil law:

In the context of not-for-profit corporations, directors' conduct constituting a tort is the case of negligent mismanagement. Negligent mismanagement arises when the injury suffered by the tort victim can be attributed to carelessness in the oversight of some aspect of the corporation's operations. It relates to situations where the board knew of, or ought to have foreseen, a systemic problem and failed to address it.

In my opinion, this scenario fit within the scope of negligent operations at Narconon Trois-Rivières where "the directors permitted an unsafe condition to exist on the corporation's property and that unsafe condition lead to a personal injury. This could constitute negligent mismanagement on the part of the directors and result in personal liability." The Trois-Rivières executives floundering around at Narconon were not really doing the job a normal executive would do anywhere else. Sure, they had titles and Post positions on the 'Org Board' chart hanging on the wall as being this and that. One higher up executive had more authority over the other, but it was all smoke and mirrors. These Narconon executive directors were a disgrace — always nattering about each other and not taking responsibility for their own negligent actions, as well as blaming others for their own mistakes. But, in my opinion, they were all guilty as sin for the human rights abuses that the Commission investigations found them accountable for. I wasn't going to let them get away with hiding the facts behind any of the non-disclosure agreements.

May 30, 2014, my birthday, I filed a lawsuit against Narconon Trois-Rivières, Church of Scientology, and individual executives at the courthouse in Montreal. The case was filed in the Small Claims division for Breach of Contract, Fair Game and Dead Agent practices attacking me online, and for part of the Quebec Human Rights Commission award for moral and punitive damages. When the case was filed, the limit was only $7,000 but increased over the next year to a maximum $15,000 and the court documents were amended to the increase.

In the Small Claims division, the plaintiff and defendants are not allowed to be represented by a lawyer in the courtroom — only the opposing parties, the judge, and the court clerk, will be hashing out the facts. To date, there has not been one Narconon case out of dozens filed, that have made it to a courtroom trial — all have been settled out of court or on courtroom steps at the last hour. Setting a case precedent against Narconon with evidence documents piled up for review by other lawyers, could create a domino effect for current and future cases. With Narconon executives 'gift for foot-in-mouth', I dare say I'm looking forward to facing off against the plaintiffs when, or if, this case makes it to trial.

Human Rights Commission Verdict

Even if this case isn't presented to a judge in Montreal, all of my efforts to have Scientology's Narconon human rights abuses exposed in the media and public eye, were worth every minute of the countless hours of work.

Chapter 27
Say No to Narconon at Trout Run

> We need our people and families to unite ... to question with boldness without wavering and stand tall. After all, isn't that what our Founding Fathers expected 'We the people' to do? — Barbara Post-Askin

Scientology's drug rehab centers were floundering around like a mutating virus being spewed about by someone in power who just wouldn't take no for an answer. Narconon centers in Trois-Rivières, Calgary, Georgia, and elsewhere were forced to close for various reasons including human rights abuses and fraud. Other Narconons, like Narconon Arrowhead, Scientology's flag-ship center, was only running at a fraction of their capacity. The word was out, the media, google searches, and the public could easily search and see that these cult rehabs were dangerous and deadly — some patients dying inside the centers.

New centers started using names other than Narconon, like, 'Sunshine Summit Lodge' and 'Rainbow Canyon Retreat' or 'Fresh Start Nevada' to help people not discover that these centers were in fact, Narconon. Even some of the websites do not mention the word Narconon, and especially not Scientology. The Narconon word has become like poison, and rightfully so considering at least 12 patients have died while receiving so-called treatment — and countless more relapsing or dying soon after they leave.

Now, Scientology is working very hard to pressure IAS (International Association of Scientologists) members to donate to David Miscavige's new Ideal Narconons. Some are called 'Ideal Continental Narconons' that allegedly are being created to serve the elite, well-off addicts or celebrities.

Dante's Eighth Circle

One of these 'Ideal Narconons' was called the 'DC Narconon' — giving it stature and a presence in the Washington DC area where Scientology's 'Founding Church' is located.

But the DC Narconon is not located in the District of Columbia, Washington area — it's actually located in Frederick, Maryland, at a property called, Trout Run. The property was purchased by a Scientology entity, 'Social Betterment Properties International' (SBPI) — a front group that also purchased properties in Canada and Australia for the same reason. The Trout Run property in Frederick cost nearly six million dollars, and in need of extensive repairs, renovations, and septic before a Narconon center could open.

As is often the case with Scientology ventures, they 'put the cart before the horse' in all three countries, buying the proposed drug rehab sites that were not zoned for drug rehab treatment facilities. To get around this flub, instead of calling the centers "drug rehab treatment centers" — they claimed they were only small 'Group Homes' to slide in through the bylaw back doors.

In Frederick, SBPI applied to have the Trout Run property designated as 'historic' — thinking this would allow a group home to operate under the correct zoning. Little did Scientology know they would face fierce opposition from citizens that formed a group on Facebook called, "No Narconon at Trout Run" — with a team of over 350 dedicated members. SBPI hired a lawyer and presented a lame case to the Frederick council members, bringing in Sylvia Stanard from Scientology's DC 'Office of National Affairs' and Yvonne Rodgers, Narconon's East Coast Executive Director. Of course, and as expected, an ex-Narconon graduate student was brought in to present their glowing story about how successful the Narconon program was and how it saved their life.

On the other side was a group of citizens who opposed Narconon and presented their case to council members. With the Trout Run property being close to Camp David, one person suggested to council that there could be security risks. Another gave multiple scenarios of police, ambulance, hospitals, and social services being overburdened due to 911 calls for help, and patients who were kicked out roaming the community streets.

About mid-April, 2015, I joined the Facebook group and began getting to know some in the group who were very pro-active in their 'No Narconon

Say No to Narconon at Trout Run

at Trout Run' Facebook page. Most were researching the pitfalls of the notorious drug rehab center, and educating themselves in all aspects of the cult's operations and the back-door loophole that Frederick council members were considering.

I left Montreal and flew to North Carolina where I spent a few days until Cheryl and I left for Washington DC so I could do some filming of the DC Founding Church, and of course I wanted to see the White House. After a few hours, we left for Frederick, Maryland to stay with a couple out in a rural farm area — parking the car so that 'anyone' passing by could not see we were there. I was pretty sure that Scientology's intelligence organization, Office of Special Affairs, already were aware of my visit, and I was right.

On May 11, 2015, a New York Times reporter, Andrew Siddons, contacted me for an interview about Scientology's push into Frederick. I was scheduled to give a speech to a group of concerned, Frederick citizens on May 12th at the local library. I met with the New York Times reporter for about forty minutes before the meeting. Siddons and his photographer stayed for the speech and took photos for the 'Times' newspaper.

Someone from the group noticed a car circling around out in the library parking lot looking at license plate numbers and wrote down the suspicious car plate number — taking photos of the car and person. Reporter Sylvia Carignan from the 'Frederick News-Post' and Times reporter Andrew Siddons was inside the library.

After the meeting, it was like a 'cat and mouse game' — being followed for several miles around the country side of Frederick. I had been followed on several occasions in the past, and didn't pay too much attention because I wasn't sure if we were being followed or not? I was in one car with Cheryl and we were following the car in front of us back to the farm house. I could see head-lights way back in the distance come over a crest in the road but thought it was too far away to be following us. I was unaware that the person in the car we were behind, had circled around, and was filming and taking photos with his camera of the chase.

Apparently, the same car that was circling the library parking lot was the same one following us after the meeting, and it was not just one car but two.

The following is a narrative from a group member at the meeting.

Dante's Eighth Circle

May 12, 2015 — Scientology dirty tricks — "No Narconon at Trout Run hosted its first of two community meetings at the Urbana Regional Library from 6:00 PM to 8:00 PM

Prior to the start of the press event and community meeting, Narconon/Church of Scientology personnel distributed Narconon pamphlets at the Urbana Regional Library.

Guest speaker David E. Love was interviewed by The Washington Post and The New York Times from approximately 5:00 PM to 6:00 PM.

Attendees noticed a silver Hyundai with Virginia plates WVZ 8930 circling the Urbana Regional Library from 5:15-5:35. The car would circle the facility, stop and park for a few minutes, then circle and park again in a different spot. This pattern continued in both upper and lower parking lots. Attendees began to follow the vehicle. At this point the vehicle sped out of the lower parking lot onto Amelung Street. It then went through the roundabout onto Spring Street and picked up Urbana Pike. At this point, the vehicle speedily exited onto 270 North.

The community meeting lasted from 6:10 PM to 7:50 PM. The Frederick News-Post was at the meeting.

As it got dark, a member left the community meeting at approximately 8:20 PM and proceeded to drive north on I-270 and then north on Route 15. Guest speaker David Love was following the NN@TR member's vehicle. The NN@TR driver was alert in knowing that Narconon/Church of Scientology may follow the two vehicles based on their confirmed presence at the Urbana Regional Library when they distributed "The Narconon Program" brochure as well as the earlier incident at 5:35 PM in the parking lot. Love also communicated he had been harassed and followed by Narconon/Church of Scientology after similar events in other cities and countries he has visited.

The NN@TR driver, still on Route 15, decided to stay behind a truck that was moving at approximately 55 mph. The driver maintained this speed knowing that most cars on this stretch of Route 15 will pass a vehicle driving at that "low" speed. Several cars passed, but two cars stayed far behind in the same lane.

The NN@TR driver decided to turn off of Route 15 and head east on Biggs Ford Road, knowing few people use Biggs Ford Road at that time of night. The NN@TR driver also thought it would be conspicuous if a vehicle(s) immediately turned off Route 15. However, the two tailing vehicles turned off Route 15 and headed east on Biggs Ford Road following the NN@TR driver's car.

The NN@TR driver turned south on Fountain Rock Road, with Love following behind. Both tailing vehicles turned on Fountain Rock Road.

The NN@TR driver turned west onto Retreat Road, knowing it to be isolated and that it loops back to Biggs Ford Road. One of the following cars passed the Retreat Road turn, the tailing vehicle turned onto Retreat Road. It stopped hastily and then backed out. The NN@TR driver continued, still leading Love, until they were out of sight near the railroad tracks. They stopped and conversed, deciding to double-back to Fountain Rock Road.

Upon arrival at Fountain Rock Road, the driver saw the other tailing vehicle sitting off the road. It was to the south at the bend in Fountain Rock Road, sitting off the right shoulder with its lights on facing a position perpendicular to the road.

The NN@TR driver turned toward the tailing vehicle, accelerated fast, and flipped on high beams. The tailing vehicle pulled out heading south on Fountain Rock Road swiftly, heading toward Route 194. The NN@TR driver caught up to the vehicle as it stopped at Route 194 at approximately 8:51 PM. The NN@TR driver identified the tailing vehicle as a tan Toyota Sienna Symphony with Virginia license plate WMC-3388.

In time, the NN@TR driver and Love made it safely to their destination.

Upon arrival, the NN@TR driver compared photos taken before the community meeting at the Urbana Regional Library began with photos taken during this incident.

The NN@TR driver found evidence that the tailing tan Toyota Sienna was at the Urbana Regional Library throughout the course of the evening and had, in fact, attempted to tail the vehicle and guest speaker David Love.

Four NN@TR members along with guest speaker David E. Love drove along Catoctin Hollow Road. They were walking along the public road, admiring the stream, and talking about the impacts of a Narconon/Church of Scientology facility upon the area.

Ten minutes after being present in the area, four Frederick County Sheriff's Deputy Cruisers pulled up along the road. The NN@TR members used this time to inform the officers about their reason for being on the public road.

David E. Love showed his press credential to the officers. Other members indicated that they lived around the immediate area. It was established that the group was clearly not trespassing.

The lead officer indicated that the phone call came from "the owner" who described the NN@TR members as the online hacker/activist group Anonymous, a known entity who supports exposing Narconon/Church of Scientology.

The lead officer indicated that the person who called the police wanted the members to sign a form stating that they've been warned not to trespass. David E. Love called his lawyer. The members were respectful with the officers, but refused to sign a Letter of Trespass Notification. The members indicated to the officers that they will only give their personal information to Sheriff Chuck Jenkins.

At this point, the lead officer went through the front gate and spoke to a man inside the facility who was sitting in a black car. Members demanded to know this individual's his personal information. It was at this point that the man in the black car dropped the request for the NN@TR members to sign the letter of Trespass Notification.

NN@TR members explained how they were followed from Urbana to northern Frederick County on 5/13/15. They indicated to the responding officers that they notified the authorities of this.

The officers waited down the road to give the NN@TR members a friendly escort away from the property to be sure that they were not followed by Narconon/Church of Scientology.

'No Narconon at Trout Run' hosted its second of two community meetings at Cafe 611 from 6:00 PM to 8:00 PM.

This round of attempted harassment and intimidation from Scientology thugs was, as usual, a fail and unnecessary expense to taxpayers. It amazes me how stupid the command lines are in this cult. By making the same mistakes over and over again that cause them so much bad PR, one would think that they would finally learn. But, to no avail, the *foot bullets* and *foot-in-mouth* continues on as per L. Ron Hubbard policy. "Always attack — never defend." Scientology will never win … good always wins over evil deeds no matter what this cult tries to do or what their 'Miscavige Minions' say to media and post on Dead Agent websites. As most cults are, so is Scientology: it is a group of mind controlled, brain-washed, and indoctrinated victims. The leader, David Miscavige, is in my opinion and the opinion of many others, a paranoid coward that fears media interviews. Instead, Miscavige will have his spokesperson (Karin Pouw) usually reply with a statement in the form of a letter — most likely dictated or approved by the "Black-Hearted" Pope.

The Decision

On June 2, 2015, The Washington Post published:

> Frederick Council rejects historic designation for Trout Run, a blow for a Scientology-backed drug rehab" — Frederick County Council voted overwhelmingly Tuesday against a historical designation for Trout Run, dealing a stunning setback to a Scientology-backed drug treatment program that wants to open at the rural retreat near Camp David.
>
> The council voted 6:1 against the designation, with at least one member who had previously indicated some support for the project apparently changing sides. A large group of activists opposed to Narconon broke out into applause.
>
> One Anonymous source from Why We Protest commented that:
>
> This could turn into another Vietnam for the cult if Miscavige chooses to fight in court. I think a lawsuit would come across as vindictive and frivolous, so would create 'bad PR' as Hubbard put it. Even if two 'members' caved in, a re-vote would still maintain the status quo and the Miscavige REIT would have a piece of property they could only sell. In the years I have observed Scientology, I have never seen the

cult so agitated.

Narconon in Canada Rejected

On June 20, 2015, Scientology's appeal case to open Narconon in Ontario was dismissed. As Scientology and Narconon is well known for, they brought in non-expert witnesses, including a program graduate, appearing in support of the Narconon program. All three spoke glowingly of Narconon, but none of these witnesses addressed the land use planning matters. The Board stated:

> While the Board appreciates the time and effort these three individuals took to travel some distance to appear at this hearing, the Board attaches no weight to their evidence.

Mr. Chung and Ms. Dion testified extensively on the Narconon program including treatment and rehabilitation phases. Ms. Dion appeared to be taking the Board on a *red herring* ride with the license agreement between Narconon International and Narconon Incorporated — stating that: "Narconon International had the right of entry and inspection to ensure standards are maintained." When pressed under cross-examination, the pretense of "inspections and to ensure standards" fell apart and was exposed as false and misleading. Ms. Dion failed to explain that the entire agreement and the purpose of the right of entry and inspection is to ensure that Narconon Inc. is using properly the Narconon trademarks.

Scientology dictator, David Miscavige, failed to have 'Ideal Continental Narconons' in Canada, USA, and Australia — a huge loss and disgrace. Mike Rinder, a high ranking ex-Scientologist, stated on Tony Ortega's blog that: "Miscavige will treat it [being voted down] as an insult and he doesn't take kindly to being insulted."

Being denied and rejected, indeed, must be frustrating for Scientology and their 'Expansion Committee.' Governments, health agencies, and the public are now well aware of these dangerous drug rehab centers directed and operated by a cult organization. Too many wrongful deaths and fraud lawsuits, now totalling over thirty cases, detail how fraudulent and deadly Narconon really is.

I was visiting a grave in Oklahoma of a girl who died inside Narconon and later met a man. He was her father. On Father's Day, 2015, Murphy Robert Murphy gave expressed, written permission to quote his comment he made on Facebook.

> Today is Father's Day but I won't be hearing Happy Father's Day from my daughter Stacy Dawn Murphy. Why? Because she died at that Scientology recruitment center NarCONon — if you run across anyone in favor of a NarCONon be very concerned. In my opinion they are dishonest, self- serving or plain ignorant of the truth. Please do not allow a NarCONon into your community. Addicts seeking professional help won't get it there.

Chapter 28
Full Circle: Love versus Goliath

You can fool some of the people all of the time, and all of the people some of the time, but you cannot fool all of the people all of the time. — Abraham Lincoln

In my sincere opinion, 'Dante's Eighth Circle' represents the fraudulent seducers and liars of two-headed hypocrites. Scientology's leader, David Miscavige, their dirty tricks 'Office of Special Affairs' and the Narconon hierarchy — all work in concert in an evil attempt to control people by deception.

When I escaped from Narconon in Quebec, I had no idea how big this 'Goliath-Giant' was. And even if I had known, I doubt I would have walked away. To the contrary, the more I learned, the deeper I dug in, researched, and tapped away on my keyboard. Knowing what I know today, indeed I would have done a few things differently, but not much.

Before I complete the 'Full Circle' and finish this last chapter, Dante's 'Ninth Circle' reminds me of the captured 'Galactic Confederacy' aliens that L. Ron Hubbard mentions in the story about Xenu. Hubbard spun an interesting tail of psychiatrists gathering billions of 'Galactic' citizens — then froze them in a mixture of alcohol and glycol to capture their souls. This scenario somewhat reflects the ninth circle of hell... treachery.

When I think about David Miscavige and what appears to be his callous disregard for human rights, human dignity, and compassion for humanity as a whole, I am appalled. Who would, or could, allow their own father to die of what seemed like a heart attack without care? Who could send their own wife away for several years? Who could send top Scientology executives to Scientology's private prison — the RPF and allegedly beat these same staff members? In my opinion, there may be a special place in hell for David Miscavige — similar to Dante's ninth circle, a place called 'Caina' where souls who were traitors to their family are doomed. These souls are buried in ice which goes up to their faces.

In my opinion, David Miscavige is nothing more than a coward that uses his minion spokespersons to issue written statements to the media, name-calling critics as bigots, and being guilty of hate crimes and discrimination. Miscavige refuses to be interviewed by any media. As far as I am aware, the only time Scientology's leader was ever on camera, was with Ted Koppel on ABC News Nightline February 14, 1992. Koppel asked Miscavige direct questions that most people would find easy to answer with a simple yes or no, but not Miscavige. He stumbled through the 55 minute interview, and appeared to make a fool of himself. From that time on, Miscavige used others to go in front of media cameras.

It's obvious to many that Miscavige is a paranoid sociopath — one who pays hundreds of thousands to have ex-Scientologists, critics, media, and even his own father, followed and harassed. Two men were allegedly paid $10,000 a week to spy on David Miscavige's father, Ron Miscavige Sr. The two told police in 2013 that they were once watching Miscavige Sr. one day when he hunched over and grabbed his chest — looking to be in pain and feared that he was having a heart attack.

The two men, according to a police report, contacted David Miscavige who allegedly told them not to call for help. "If he dies, he dies. Don't intervene," David allegedly ordered. Unfortunately for his son David, Ron Miscavige Sr. lived — he was only fumbling with his phone, not a heart attack. Now Ron has a book deal with a major publisher about Scientology, titled: "If He Dies, He Dies."

When I read this story, I found it difficult to believe or understand how a person could be so callous. In my mind, I compared David Miscavige to cult leader, Jim Jones, who led more than 900 followers in a mass suicide known as the Jonestown Massacre. Not that I think Miscavige would or could do the same, only that he acts and behaves similar at times, seeking to control and micromanage attacks on critics and the unfaithful.

Scientology, Miscavige, and Narconon executives truly believe that I am a so-called 'Suppressive Person' — having an 'anti-social personality', impeding the progress of Scientology and their Narconons. Apparently, the reason I'm looked upon as being a danger, is because those around or connected to me become 'Potential Trouble Sources'. According to Scientology, "The anti-social personality supports only destructive groups and rages against and attacks any constructive or betterment group." And: "The anti-social cannot finish a cycle of action. Such become surrounded with incomplete projects." The Suppressive Person is also known as the Anti-Social Personality.

On Scientology's own website, they state: "The basic reason the Suppressive Person behaves as he or she does lies in a hidden terror of others. To such a person every other being is an enemy, an enemy to be covertly or overtly destroyed. The fixation is that survival itself depends on "keeping others down" or "keeping people ignorant."

In my opinion, this sounds more like David Miscavige is the 'monster' Suppressive Person (SP) that describes him in detail without reservation whatsoever. Lying, hiding, and unable to finish a 'Narconon Expansion' cycle depicts an 'anti-social' personality in Scientology terms. It's quite evident that many of Miscavige's actions end in catastrophe and mayhem, resulting in bad PR and ridicule.

"Keeping people down and ignorant" defines a cult leader and evil dictator...It defines a Suppressive Person. When a cult leader is pathological or, better said, a toxic danger to others, then one can anticipate that at some point those who associate with him will likely suffer physically, emotionally, psychologically, or financially.

When examining cult leaders, the narcissist does not respect the boundaries and privacy of his reluctant adherents. He ignores their wishes and treats them as objects or instruments of gratification. He seeks to control all situations and people compulsively. He often lies to support unfounded claims like "we're expanding more than ever" and "serving more people today" claims.

Taking another step, a 'Narcissistic Sociopath' is charming, manipulative, grandiose, lying, authoritarian, secretive, and divisive...to name a few traits. Does this fit David Miscavige? In my opinion, yes, it certainly does. A narcissistic sociopath is unable to tolerate criticism and needs constant praise, as well as deference from other people. The narcissist with sociopathic traits reacts strongly and sometimes even violently to negative feedback.

Dante's Eighth Circle

The very sad thing about Scientology is that David Miscavige and his staff could help so many suffering souls — if they chose to do so. This organization has billions of dollars in their 'war-chest' to fight lawsuits and huge, untold sums in real estate holdings. This evil cult has the ability to turn 'full circle' and benefit society, especially the downtrodden and drug addicts. In not doing so, they become their own worst enemy from within, and the public sees them as a crazy cult.

They could run Narconons with professional, qualified staff. Doctors, nurses, and psychiatrists on board could treat the 'patients' with science-based therapy and treatments. Scientology could make a difference in helping hundreds of thousands. But, this will never happen. They will continue on status quo, running their Narconon drug rehab centers with quackery and junk-science. More people will die. It's not a matter of if, but when will there be another victim removed from Narconon dead.

Scientology does not deserve an IRS tax exempt status in the USA. This so-called charity is a fail when defining a 'public benefit' — pathetic and disgusting. The Church of Scientology and its front groups like Narconon are engaged in systematic violations of the terms of their tax exemption.

Scientology was not given tax exemption for the purposes of paying law firms and lawyers to hire private investigators. Especially when the purposes are for acts of spying, harassment, and intimidation. These attacks continue on today against ex-Scientologists, critics, journalists, and media who expose Scientology abuses. This is Scientology policy — to attack, and destroy all of these people. "Never defend, always attack."

I expect to be attacked again by Scientology because of this book. They will likely say I'm a bigot filled with hate, and an "anti-Scientology extremist" as published on a *Scientology Myths* website. But this is not the case whatsoever. This book was not written to attack, rather to expose the lies and fraud inside Scientology and Narconon. I don't 'hate' David Miscavige, his executives, or the Narconon hierarchy. What I do hate is their abusive, deadly actions and behaviour.

David Miscavige may rule with a tiny fist, but his control over Scientology members and their front groups like Narconon, are under his direction and spell. When you look at the dictator of a cult group, look at how the organization operates and the signature of fraud and deception attached to it. Even though the organizational directives may be hidden from sight, the organization will always bear the type of "fruit" dictated by any cult leader, such as Miscavige.

I can't remember how many times I've read all 2,800 pages of the eight Narconon books, and researched other source documents. One issue that is not mentioned often is how much money these Narconons rake in, especially the Registrars and their weekly income. I worked in adjoining offices as a Registrar with two others, three of us on the phones all day long. At Narconon Trois-Rivières, the program fee was only $23,000 but if a Registrar brings in 2 people per week, that earns them a $5,600 paycheck each week in commissions. One of the Registrars working in the office next to me closed 3-5 sales in a good week.

The Registrars were earning more than some of the executive directors. But this is where the danger lies. The potential to earn such a high income causes the Registrars to mislead, misrepresent, and lie to the patients or their sponsoring loved ones. Once the sale is closed and the patient (student) arrives with the $23,000 check in hand or a Credit Card pays the fees, good luck getting any money back. It's very rare to see any refunds or even partial refunds. Even if the patient is kicked out the first week or month, the 'Mark' has been had, and the scam succeeds again in filling Narconon and Scientology coffers.

David Miscavige can't say he knows nothing about Narconon operations or that he is not involved. He personally visited Narconon Arrowhead as seen in a group photo circulating the internet. Scientology's dirty tricks agency, Office of Special Affairs, cannot deny they are involved in Narconon. Yvette Shank, director of Canada's Office of Special Affairs and president of Scientology Canada, was at Narconon Trois-Riviers on occasion... shortly before it was closed by the Quebec health agency.

Scientology Montreal cannot deny its involvement with Narconon Trois-Rivières. Large donations were made directly from Narconon to Scientology Montreal, and a leaked email posted on WikiLeaks confirms how much control Scientology had over Narconon in Canada. This was an important document that the Quebec Human Rights Commission investigated and asked Narconon why they were seeking advice from Scientology.

Dealing with a Black Panther Operation:

De: Jean Lariviere <jean_lariviere@hotmail.com>

Objet: RUSH — URGENT — Coming bill/new law re. Narconon in Quebec in Fall of 2008

Date: Wed, 16 Jul 2008 04:14:59 +0000

A: <sylvain.fournier@narconon.ca>

CC: <marc.bernard@narconon.ca> <rejeanne.fleury@narcononcanada.ca> <aline.proulx@narconon.ca> <ablecanada@thunderstar.net> <dsaqbc-@oricom.ca> <crncarr@aol.com> <data@scientology-tor.ca>

Dear Sylvain, [Narconon Trois-Rivières Executive Director]

Over 2 months ago, yourself, Aline and I met in Montreal to go over the situation of the media attacks on Radio-Canada and other medias and the statement made by the Minister of Health on television that a new bill/law would be tabled at the Quebec legislative assembly in the Fall of 2008 to regulate or control drug detox and/or drug rehab activities such as those taking place at Narconon 3-Rivers.

My recommendation to you — based on my 25-year experience in public affairs including holding the post of DSA in the province of Quebec for over twenty years — was that NN need to first and right away — asap — establish the extent and nature of the threat or risk so that you would know asap what Narconon is facing or dealing with, and thus be in a position to then correctly estimate the situation and the extent and nature of the handling needed to properly handle the situation!

The truth was that you did/do not really know what this law is about. How can NN handle an unknown threat? Obviously, the first thing to do is to find out what this law is about, and what is the sit between NN and the Quebec governments!

For that specific purpose, I recommended that you (or someone like you who knows well NN activities and the activities of other drug rehab/detox groups in Quebec) to go right away — asap — do a few visits in Quebec City at the Ministry of Health and Social Services and meet with government officials who are overseeing the area of drug detox and drug rehab — and who are likely the guys who are writing the new law and who are making recommendations to the Minister — to find out what is the contents and extent of the law that is to come out in the Fall of 2008. Also, to do so very overtly as a NN staff so that

Full Circle: Love versus Goliath

you find out exactly what they think about NN and what needs to be handled. In other words, find out from the horse's mouth so to speak! Two (2) major targets:

1. gathering basic and essential information and;

2. starting the PR handling right away with the people who must be handled!

You agreed that was the right thing to do and you agreed it was to be done right away, asap so that you would be able to meet with them before they would go in Summer vacation... You were also supposed to let me know the results of those meetings so that I could assist with your writing a tailor-made handling or plan to handle the actual situation.

I have heard nothing from you since then so I do not know if you did any visits with the relevant officials at the Ministry of Health in Quebec City. If no such visits have been done, then it is likely that Narconon 3-Rivieres is back in the same position that it was 2 months ago... except that NN 3-Rivieres is that much closer to having to deal with a possibly very ominous situation that cannot yet be properly assessed and handled until such visits and data gathering activities are made.

Please check what LRH says about dealing with a Black Panther!

As you know NN is not the Church and the Church is not going to and cannot meet with government officials on behalf of Narconon. No Church or DSA staff can do the job for you. Either you do it or someone else at or for NN does it. In any event, it must be confronted and done. The faster it is confronted the better and the better chances NN will have to handle the situation. I can only offer advices and the above is about the best advices I can give you my friend!

I am always willing to talk with you and offer data or advices.

Best,

Jean Larivière [Director of Public Affairs Montreal]

Dante's Eighth Circle

De: Sylvain Fournier <sylvain.fournier@narconon.ca>

Objet: RE: RUSH — URGENT — Coming bill/new law re. Narconon in Quebec in Fall of 2008

Date: Wed, 23 Jul 2008 14:37:46-0400

A: <jean_lariviere@hotmail.com>

CC: <marc.bernard@narconon.ca> <rejeanne.fleury@narcononcanada.ca> <aline.proulx@narconon.ca> <ablecanada@thunderstar.net> <dsaqbc-@oricom.ca> <crncarr@aol.com> <data@scientology-tor.ca>

Dear Jean, [Executive Director Narconon Trois-Rivières]

Thank you for your communication, and for your advice throughout this episode, I did use a lot of your recommendation to handle this situation.

You proposed to me: establish the extent and nature of the threat or risk so that you would know asap what Narconon is facing.

Which I did, on multiple occasions. I have a very good communication line with the Office of M. Sebastion Proulx, who is the Deputy of the Mauricie Region, which includes Trois-Rivières, he is also the Official Opposition House Leader and Official Opposition critic for education.

On top of that he is also the right-hand man of M. Dumont who is the leader of the Official Opposition at the Quebec Parliament.

M.Proulx does obviously sit at the Parliament of Quebec.

Every time I met with the deputy or his representative, I asked them if something was coming, any change at the parliament or any new law was about to be proposed or voted, or any talks about the accreditation for drug rehab; Is the accreditation's going to be mandatory ? Is the governement going to do any change about the already established accreditation ?

Each and every time they told me that nothing was going on, no change whatsoever, no new laws, no enforcement of the accreditation, nothing on the agenda at the parliament on that matter neither.

So, there is apparently no threat or risk, change or proposition to control drug rehab and NN Trois-Rivières of any form (as of 2 weeks ago).

Full Circle: Love versus Goliath

On top of that, as you probably know, the former Minister of Health and Social Services, that did make a statement on Radio-Canada, M. Phillipe Couillard, is no longer on post, he gave his resignation about a month ago. the New Minister of Health and Social Services apparently has a new agenda and drug rehabilitation is not one of his mandate, or at least not something he wants to work on. I got these information from the representative of M.Proulx himself about 2 weeks ago.

To my knowledge there is no more threat pending on top of Narconon Trois-Rivières head. I keep my eyes and ears open and talk with the Representatives of the Office of M.Proulx regularly.

We will keep applying FLORISH AND PROSPER and the enemy will fall into apathy, just like M.Couillard giving his resignation from one of the most powerful post you can have at the Parliament !!!

I will keep you updated on any future communication that I will have with M.Proulx's office, so that you are in the know.

I will most likely meet with them next week-end (26-27 July) and the 4th of September, both time on occasion where Narconon Trois-Rivières is the Major Sponsor of a large scale event (Le Monaco and Pro-Am Golf Tournament for Interval).

Thank you for your time, help and consideration.

Sylvain Fournier, *C.C.D.C. [Executive Director Narconon Trois-Rivières]
*Certified Chemical Dependency Counselor

Senior Director for Expansion
Legal Officer
Narconon Trois-Rivières
819-376-8181 ext.320 (office)
819-███████ (cell)
sylvain.fournier@narconon.ca
web:www.narconon.ca

This email clearly depicts Scientology hovering over Narconon Trois-Rivières and demanding that:

> NN need to first and right away — asap — establish the extent and nature of the threat or risk so that you would know asap what Narconon is facing or dealing with, and thus be in a position to then correctly

estimate the situation and the extent and nature of the handling needed to properly handle the situation!

In other words, find out from the horse's mouth so to speak! Two (2) major targets:

1. gathering basic and essential information and;
2. starting the PR handling right away with the people who must be handled!

Then, Jean Lariviere details how much Scientology is involved:

You were also supposed to let me know the results of those meetings so that I could assist with your writing a tailor-made handling or plan to handle the actual situation. The faster it is confronted the better and the better chances NN will have to handle the situation. I can only offer advices and the above is about the best advices I can give you my friend!

Narconon executive director, Sylvain Fournier, cowers in obedience:

I will keep you updated on any future communication that I will have with M.Proulx's office, so that you are in the know. Thank you for your time, help and consideration.

Sylvain Fournier signed his email with:

*C.C.D.C. [Executive Director Narconon Trois-Rivières]
*Certified Chemical Dependency Counselor.

How much fraud and deception could there be in the Narconon drug rehab network? Sylvain Fournier promoted and advertised himself to be a Certified Chemical Dependency Counselor (CCDC) on websites. It turned out to be a fraudulent claim and Sylvain Fournier, Narconon Trois-Riviers, David Miscavige, and approximately eighty additional respondents had a massive lawsuit filed against them.

The National Association of Forensic Counselors (NAFC) filed the lawsuit alleging Narconon employees were obtaining their certifications as Certified

Chemical Dependency Counselors through fraudulent means, and "Misuse of NAFC Mark, Certifications and Logos."

The 'Causes of Action' claimed Federal Trademark Infringement, Common Law Trademark Infringement, Federal Infringement, Violation Of Right Of Publicity, Civil Conspiracy, and a Request For Injunction against all defendants to refrain from using NAFC Certifications and/or Logo that are the subject of this litigation.

Scientology's Narconon rehab centers are indeed a cash cow for this cult of fraud, and it appears they believe they can operate above the laws of the land. What I have witnessed and experienced over the past few years, reveals an organization that has tunnel vision only for the almighty dollar. The collateral damage and suffering to victims who fall by the wayside are of no concern.

Indeed, Scientology is a Goliath of untold wealth, and they do have a right to believe what they want. But, as Senator Nicholas Xenophon stated, "There are limits on how you can behave. It's called the law, and no one is above it."

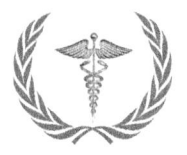

Acknowledgements

With love and respect, I am very grateful to all who contributed to this book. I am also indebted to all those who generously gave me their support, encouragement and inspiration over the past five years.

I hope I have been able to give some insight into what I and others endured. I am honored to have crossed paths with many of the students at Narconon and to this day, think of them often with warm thoughts and love. If it wasn't for our close connections, I may not have survived to see this book come to fruition. I believe that we will never give up or say that we can't do something, or that something seems impossible. No matter how discouraging each step appears, we are only limited by what we allow ourselves to be.

No matter what we've been through, we're still here. Even though the past may have hurt, betrayed, and abused, we are never defeated unless we give up. I hope we all will continue to press on with success and victory, transforming ourselves from victim to survivor. Many thanks to all who never gave up on me and stood by me. It is my sincere belief and hope that there will be justice for all those who suffered. Bless you all.

— David E. Love

References

[1] Dante Alighieri and translated by John D. Sinclair. *Inferno: The Divine Comedy, Vol. 1.* Oxford University Press, New York, NY, 1961.

[2] Jon Atack. *A Piece of Blue Sky : Scientology, Dianetics, and L. Ron Hubbard exposed.* Carol Pub. Group, New York, NY, 1990.

[3] Richard Behar. The Thriving Cult of Greed and Power. *Time Magazine*, pages 50+, Cover Story, May 1991.

[4] Lucas Aaron Catton. *Have You Told All? : Inside My Time with Narconon and Scientology.* Catton, United States, 2013.

[5] John Duignan. *The Complex: An Insider Exposes the Covert World of the Church of Scientology.* Merlin Publishing, Ireland, 2008.

[6] *Booski* from Ireland. Narconon's fishing emails, 2014.

[7] Narconon Exposed. Research website, 2002.

[8] Jefferson Hawkins. *Counterfeit Dreams.* Hawkeye Publ. Co., United States, 2010.

[9] Jefferson Hawkins. *Leaving Scientology: A Practical Guide to Escape and Recovery.* Hawkeye Publ., United States, 2012.

[10] Jefferson Hawkins. *Closing Minds: How Scientology's 'Ethics Technology' is Used to Control Their Members.* Hawkeye Publ., United States, 2015.

[11] Mark Headley. *Blown for Good — Behind the Iron Curtain of Scientology.* BFG Books, United States, 2009.

[12] Jenna Miscavige Hill. *Beyond Belief.* Harper Collins, New York, NY, 2013.

[13] Nancy Many. *My Billion Year Contract: Memoir of a Former Scientologist.* CNM Publ., United States, 2009.

[14] Russel Miller. *Bare-faced Messiah.* Michael Joseph, London, 1987.

[15] Tony Ortega. *The Unbreakable Miss Lovely: How the Church of Scientology Tried to Destroy Paulette Cooper.* Silvertail Books, London, 2015.

[16] Robert Vincent Piro. *When God Called On My Cellphone.* Xlibris Corp, Bloomington, IN, 2011.

[17] Mark 'Marty' Rathbun. *Memoirs of a Scientology Warrior.* Rathbun, United States, 2013.

[18] (RFTTP) Reaching For The Tipping Point. Research website, 2015.

[19] Janet Reitman. *Inside Scientology.* Houghton Mifflin Harcourt Publ. Co., United States, 2011.

[20] Narconon Reviews. Research website, 2013.

[21] Amy Scobee. *Scientology — Abuse At the Top.* Scobee Publ., Puyallup, WA, 2010.

[22] John Sweeney. *The Church of Fear: Inside The Weird World of Scientology.* Silvertail Books, United Kingdom, 2013.

[23] Lawrence Wright. *Going Clear.* Vintage, New York, NY, 2013.

Scientology Glossary

aberrated: Hubbard's term for derangement or insanity. "The wog world is heavily aberrated."

affinity: Used as a synonym for love or like.

affluence: A condition or level of high and climbing production. Aptly named, as higher production means more money. "The stats will be in screaming affluence again this Thursday at 2:00 p."

analytical mind: The thinking, computing mind; term used chiefly in Dianetics.

auditing: Resembling a blend of confession, psychotherapy, and hypnosis, auditing is one of the central practices of Scientology, intended to increase a person's self-knowledge and remove emotional barriers tied to past experiences. An auditor asks the person being audited sets of questions directed at uncovering subconscious memories believed to be the root of trauma, addiction, or other obstructions to happy, ethical living. Auditing is an integral part of advancement in the ranks of Scientology. The contents of auditing sessions are said to be confidential, except in cases where the church has reportedly allowed them to be used to blackmail disaffected members.

blow: To leave the church.

Cal-Mag: Cal-Mag is a soluable calcium and magnesium salt mix in a vinegar solution that L. Ron Hubbard proscribes for people doing the Purification Rundown in Scientology. Hubbard claims in his issues on the Purif that Cal-Mag prevents muscle spasms and aches. In Scientology, it is advocated as a relaxant.

charge: Mental mass in restimulation, or constant upheaval, contained in the reactive mind, or memory bank. This may not make much sense, but then, many things in Scientology are like that. In colloquial usage, charge refers to areas a person may be touchy about.

clear: A church follower who has reached the first of two main levels on the way to salvation, after undergoing auditing and freeing himself from the negative influence of his subconscious (see Reactive Mind). Before becoming a Clear, converts are known as "pre-clears."

dead agent: A verb, meaning to slander a person or disprove a piece of information to such an extent that he or it can never be used against you. "We need to dead agent that article."

declared, to be declared: To be labelled a Suppressive Person (evil) and thrown out of Scientology. People who are declared may not have *any contact* with Scientologists, and Scientologists can be declared for talking to a declared person.

degraded being: Someone so infested with body thetans, evil spirits, as to be in-auditable or insane. Also used as a general derogatory term. "These psychs are all DBs; without the tech, they won't make it."

Dianetics: The name for the theories of L. Ron Hubbard, the founder of Scientology. Hubbard described Dianetics as "a spiritual-healing technology" and an "organized science of thought," though it is overwhelmingly seen in the scientific community as pseudoscience. The purpose of Dianetics is to overcome the subconscious, which Scientologists believe is responsible for problems in physical, mental, and moral health.

disconnection: One of the most controversial practices of Scientology, in which converts are required to sever ties with all friends and family members believed to be unsupportive of their decision to join the church. Those hostile to the church — including members who become skeptical — may be labelled a "suppressive person," forcing other Scientologists to shun them. (See Suppressive Person).

e-meter: An electronic device created in the 1940s by Volney Mathison, an inventor and early collaborator with L. Ron Hubbard. E-meters are used during auditing sessions to measure the electrical conductance of a person's skin, which Scientologists believe indicates changes in the "reactive mind" of the person being audited. Hubbard claimed that E-meters were sensitive enough to detect the screams of fruit being sliced. Mathison later became disillusioned with Hubbard and his theories and criticized the use of the E-meter by the Scientology leader and others for their "phony systems." E-meter prices range from under $100 to more than $1,000 and up.

engram: A hypothetical process by which memories are claimed to be recorded in the brain — something still researched and speculated about in modern science. In the teachings of Dianetics, the engram is described as a mental picture, a recording of an experience that contained pain and some type of threat to a person's survival. Discovered through auditing, a person's engrams supposedly fit together to form a time track.

entheta: Something negative. Sad emotions, bad news, an angry letter, a violent movie — all of these things can be said to be "entheta".

Fair Game: Scientology's policy of retaliating against perceived enemies, based on Hubbard's writing that "suppressive persons" may be "deprived of property or injured by any means by any Scientologist ... May be tricked, sued, or lied to, or destroyed." Hubbard later cancelled this order because it created bad PR, but the church has continued to follow it, resulting in its reputation for litigation. The church has also carried out numerous harassment campaigns against ex-members and critics. In the most famous case, known as Operation Freakout, the FBI discovered that the church had harassed, threatened, and plotted against journalist Paulette Cooper with an elaborate scheme to have her imprisoned or placed in a mental institution. More recently, the church tried to destroy the business of a man who employed a high-ranking defector.

Gold Base: The international headquarters of the Church of Scientology in Riverside County, Calif. Gold Base is a 700-acre compound whose location was kept secret even from lower-level Scientologists until the last decade. It is the home of Scientology's top officials and the headquarters of the Sea Org.

Non-Enturbulation Order: An order issued to you if you are very close to being thrown out. The order basically warns you that if you upset anyone else, or if the ethics officer receives any bad reports about you, you will be in serious trouble.

O/Ws: Overts and Withholds, which essentially means sins and secrets.

Office of Special Affairs: Officially the branch responsible for Scientology's legal affairs and public relations, the Office of Special Affairs has drawn considerable attention for acting as the church's "secret police," carrying out "dead agent" or "Fair Game" operations against the church's enemies. Other plots involved the OSA attempting to frame targets for phony crimes.

Operating Thetan: a Scientologist who has reached the second level in the religion's hierarchy of salvation. The designation is divided into eight sublevels, which gradually reveal the deepest secrets of the church, including its creation story, which is revealed in the infamous OT III. According to ex-Scientologists and investigative reporters, progressing through the final echelons costs tens of thousands of dollars. Tom Cruise is rumoured to be an OT VII.

out tech: Diverging from what Scientologists believe is "standard" Hubbard doctrine.

PTS/SP (course): A major Scientology course in which one's learns Hubbard's thoughts on evil people, and how to deal with them, and what happens when one is connected to an evil person. See also: Potential Trouble Source, Suppressive Person

Potential Trouble Source (or PTS): Someone who is connected to a Suppressive Person (SP). According to Scientology a PTS will often be sick (in fact, they believe that PTSness is the only reason anyone gets sick), have emotional ups and downs, and not be able to get very far in life.

RPF: Rehabilitation Project Force. When a Sea Org member has done something considered particularly bad, they are isolated from the rest of the Sea Org members in the RPF program. People on the RPF are not allowed to walk (they run everywhere), are not allowed to speak to another Sea Org member unless spoken to, and spend most of their time doing manual labour. This is a very controversial program. Scientologists call it "rehabilitation", critics call it "slave labour".

raw meat: Someone who just joined Scientology, or is thinking about joining Scientology. This is commonly used among the staff and Sea Org members, but not really among the public.

reactive mind: The subconscious half of the human mind containing a person's involuntary impulses. (The conscious mind is known as the analytic mind.) The goal of auditing and most other Scientology practices is to abolish the reactive mind, which Hubbard believed was the cause of most people's physical and mental problems.

Reg: Someone responsible for raising money for the org. Can also be used as a verb, eg. "She was regging money."

Sea Org: A fraternal order that originated from Hubbard's sea travels in the 1960s, when he invented the upper levels of Scientology. Sea Org members, some of whom are teenagers, sign contracts for up to a billion years of service, and are discouraged from having families of their own. The organization has drawn fire for drafting Scientologist children before they are 18 years old, sequestering them from mainstream life in compounds and aboard the Freewinds, and according to some ex-members, held prisoner and required to do forced labour. Katie Holmes's exit from the church is rumoured to be driven by her fear that her daughter, Suri, was being groomed for the Sea Org.

stats: Statistics. Most Scientology staff members, Sea Org members, business persons and school children keep statistics of their work and progress in order to measure their production. See also: upstat, downstat.

suppressive person: Officially, a person with sociopathic tendencies or behaviours. In practice, the label is a catch-all term that church leadership uses for anyone at odds with Scientology, including internal critics. Since church teaching forbids members from associating with SPs, parents may be required to kick their kids out of the house or spouses to cease contact with each other. The term originates from Scientology's growth in the 1960s, when Hubbard intensified his authoritarian control of the movement. Even he, however, expressed concern that the church was abusing the label with an overly elastic definition.

TRs: Training Routines. These are basic drills done in Scientology meant to improve your communication skills. These include TR0, wherein two students sit across from each other with their eyes closed with the purpose of learning to "be there comfortably", and TR0 Bullbait, wherein one student must sit perfectly still while another yells, screams, tells jokes, or in any other way tries to get him/her to react.

thetan: an invisible part of a human being, similar to the concept of a soul or spirit in other religions, that exists whether or not it is currently operating a human body. Scientologists believe Thetans are trillions of years old, having been reborn repeatedly in various earthly bodies. They are responsible for the existence of the material world, which they willed into being, according to Dianetics.

Twin: A course partner. Twins study everything on any particular course together, and help each other through the course. You can also say you are "twinning" with someone.

verbal tech: Talking about Scientology doctrine, debating about Scientology doctrine, or discussing Scientology doctrine without physically referencing the applicable text. Hubbard was very cautious about people altering his writings from their original form, and so he forbade anyone from discussing the intricacies of Scientology without actually pulling out the appropriate book and referencing the doctrine directly. It is a high crime in Scientology to spread verbal tech.

withhold: A secret, something bad that you haven't told anyone about.

Wog: A derogatory term meaning "non-scientologist".

Xenu: According to Hubbard, the dictator of a Galactic Confederacy who brought billions of people to Earth and massacred them with hydrogen bombs 75 trillion years ago. The slaughter, known as "Incident II," sets up a major conflict in Scientology, as the thetans of the victims devolved into "body thetans" that torment modern humans. Releasing their grip is part of the goal of Scientology. The story of Xenu, which the church tried to keep secret until it leaked via an Internet newsgroup in 1994, is revealed in Operating Thetan level three, or OT III. Some Scientology officials now deny the existence of the Xenu story.

Front Cover Photo Credit: Carole Raddato, Frankfurt, Germany. *Entrance to the Cave of the Sibyl, Cumae.* (File from *Wikimedia Commons*, via *file upload bot*, Magnus Manske.)

Cover Design Collaboration: Gary Lee-Nova (Canadian Artist) with Anonymous friends at WWP and ESMB.

Editors: Cheryl E. Dickens-Harlow, with friends at *Why We Protest*

Typesetting: Typeset in Linux Libertine by a friend at *WWP*, using a MiKTeX distribution of LaTeX.

©2015 David E. Love. Complete research documents can be found online at http://smartpeopletoday.net/.